Seeing Space

Dedicated to Joanna Crone-Ravestein,
my guardian angel in later years

Seeing Space

Robert A. Crone

SWETS & ZEITLINGER
PUBLISHERS

LISSE ABINGDON EXTON (PA) TOKYO

Library of Congress Cataloging-in-Publication Data

Applied for

Typesetting: Charon Tec Pvt. Ltd, Chennai, India
Printed by: Krips, Meppel, The Netherlands

Published by: Swets & Zeitlinger Publishers
www.szp.swets.nl

ISBN 90 265 1955 9

Contents

Preface

Space, like light and colour, is a fundamental aspect of vision. A number of publications on spatial vision have been made. Most of them are concerned with details which are hardly accessible because of their high degree of specialisation in the areas of neurophysiology, systems theory, philosophy or psychology. This book aims at a brief non-specialised survey of the whole subject. I have tried to explain difficult things in a simple way, to keep the style light and to offer the reader relaxation every now and then with a historical digression. I have not given detailed information about differing points of view, but have given preference to the insights I have acquired myself as an ophthalmologist during many decennia of clinical and theoretical work. *Seeing Space* has been written for eye specialists, ophthalmic opticians, psychologists and other practitioners of visual science, and also for anyone possessing some knowledge of science who is interested in spatial vision.

The book contains three parts. Part I describes general aspects of space and spatial perception. Part II begins with a short, elementary survey of the visual system (Chapter 4). As eye movements are of crucial importance for spatial vision, the evolution of the eye and the eye movements is elaborated in Chapter 5. The specific characteristics of spatial vision, the recognition of direction, depth and movement, are treated in the other chapters of Part II. Part III describes the spatial identification of visual objects.

Acknowledgements

I am indebted to Wim van de Grind, former professor of comparative physiology in Utrecht and to Huib Simonsz, professor of ophthalmology in Rotterdam for their valuable comments. I also thank the translator Kathleen Boet-Herbert for translating my Dutch. My publisher, Swets and Zeitlinger, has helped me greatly with the editing of the manuscript.

This book is an adaptation of the chapter 'Localisation' in *Diplopia* (1973, 1993) and the chapters on spatial vision in *Licht–Kleur–Ruimte* (1992, in Dutch). Most of the illustrations have been reproduced with permission from these two sources. The author would like to acknowledge the permission to reproduce the figures which were not included in earlier work. In all cases the origin of the figure has been indicated in the legend to the figure.

Part I

1. A Short History of Space[1]

'Space' is a word that we use every day, but if anyone were to ask us what space is, it becomes apparent that it is a mystery. Space has something to do with the position of things, but exactly what the relationship is is difficult to say. We don't always mean the same thing when we say 'space.' When a billiard player says that there is space between two billiard balls which are lying close together, he obviously means what is lying *between things.* When a cancer surgeon speaks of a 'space-occupying lesion,' he means something quite different: the *measurements of the thing itself,* which is growing and threatening life. And finally, when one speaks of space travel, one thinks of space as an *infinite ocean* in which Gagarin and Armstrong have dipped their toes.

SPACE IN ANCIENT TIMES

The pre-Socratic Greek philosophers (600–400 BC) already discovered how difficult it is to say what space is. Is space the void between things which really exist? But if the void is non-existent, isn't the spatial separation only an illusion? This was the point reached by Parmenides of Elea (500 BC), who only recognized fullness, the *plenum*, as reality, and considered ultimate reality to be found in the form of a sphere (a sort of neutron star, as we should say now).

To the atomist Democritus of Abdera (400 BC) empty space was as real as matter. Reality consisted of an infinite number of atoms floating *between* infinite emptiness. How could space possibly be finite? Lucretius, the Latin poet of atomism (75 BC), put it like this: If someone stands near the end of space and throws a spear, the spear does not suddenly stop at the boundary of space. Therefore, space must be infinite. There is a striking resemblance between the atomists' ideas and those of classical physics (which owes a lot to the rehabilitation of atomism in the Renaissance). But space was something different to the ancient atomists than to Newton: it was not the surroundings in which the atoms existed, but the gaps (*diastema*) between the atoms.

Aristotle (350 BC) rejects atomism on account of his own view of the world. For Aristotle the universe is finite, with the earth at the centre. Around it are

[1] Jammer, 1954.

concentric spheres: the spheres of the moon, the sun, the planets and the fixed stars. Space has an internal structure, which causes heavy objects in the sublunary sphere to fall downwards, in the direction of their 'natural place,' the centre of the universe, and light objects, such as fire, to move in the opposite direction. In the spheres of the planets and the fixed stars, the natural direction of movement is circular. In the heavens, where other laws apply than in the sublunary sphere, there must be a different substance (not fire, water, air or earth), a fifth element, a *quinta essentia*.

Aristotle avoids the abstract idea of space and concentrates on the psychologically more accessible idea of *place*. He tries to define the place where a material object is. Naturally that isn't the object itself; the place is only incidental, an *accidens*, which really exists, but has no independent existence like a substantial body. It is the *enveloping boundary of the body.* A moving object frees itself from its old place, and takes over a new place in space. The outer sphere of the universe has no enveloping boundary, thus no place and no limit.

Aristotle is convinced that a vacuum is an impossibility and is profuse in arguments to disprove the existence of a void. An example: if material objects were in a void, nothing would be able to make them move, and if they were moving, nothing would be able to stop them; for that matter: bodies of different weights would all fall in a void at the same high speed, an assumption which was in disagreement with Aristotle's physical ideas (which did not include inertia and gravity).

Contrary to Aristotle, the Stoa, a later philosophical school, believed that an empty space did exist outside the universe. The universe did not spread into this void because it has an inner cohesion, its own tension (*tonos*). Posidonius (100 BC) discovered that the tides were caused by the moon, a strong argument for the existence of this tension. But the 'extracosmic' void could not be missed, because the world was subjected to cycles of thermic expansion and contraction. We are reminded of modern hypotheses about the 'Big Bang' and the 'Big Crunch,' but also of ideas about Perpetual Return, as found in Oriental religions, and also in Nietzsche.

SPACE THEORY IN THE MIDDLE AGES

In the Middle Ages, Judaeo-Christian theology took over space. This led to extremely difficult problems and sharply conflicting views. The Jewish philosopher Philo (25 AD) considered that space existed before the Creation as the omnipresence of God, but Augustine (400 AD) thought that God was within Himself (*in seipso*) before the first day of creation: space only existed after God had created heaven and earth. But what sort of space was it? Aristotle's finite intracosmic plenum didn't appear to offer any room for God's omnipresence. The infinite extracosmic space assumed by the Stoa, did not seem suitable either: if God is infinite and omnipresent, he can hardly create infinite space and stay out of it himself. Realization of this leads inevitably to the idea that God himself is the infinite space. This final idea led, in point of fact, to the *divinisation* of space. As long as no features, such as dimensionality, structure or content, were ascribed to God's Immensity, no theological objections to this divinisation arose.

SPACE IN THE RENAISSANCE[2]

When, in the Renaissance, Aristotle's authority began to wane, people began to wonder if nature really abhorred a vacuum. It was difficult to explain how water could be sucked upwards in a straw against its natural direction. Is the water not only obedient to its own nature (*natura particularis*) but also to a heavenly power (*virtus celestis*)? In the middle of the seventeenth century Torricelli and Pascal radically disposed of the theory of *horror vacui*.

Acquaintance with the antique atomic theory also helped to make people less afraid of a vacuum, and they began to assume that extracosmic and intracosmic space were one. This had important consequences. It was already agreed that the space in the world had a three-dimensional structure, but now the assumption was made that this was also true for infinite space. Gassendi, (1564–1642) whose opinions resembled those of Democritus and Epicurus, described space as *non-created, infinite, immovable, three-dimensional, empty and objectively existing.* He was one of the most important precursors of Newtonian science; although he was a priest, he refused to identify God with space. The English theologian Henry More (1642–1727), on the other hand, did not abandon the medieval divinisation of space and reached the radical conclusion that God is a three-dimensional being. This point of view was unacceptable for most people, almost as unacceptable as Spinoza's idea that God and nature are one (*una substantia sive deus sive natura*). Even so, Newton has been influenced by More. He says that we, human beings, only have images of things 'in our little sensoriums' but that God exercises his will 'in his boundless uniform sensorium,' the still divinised absolute space.

NEWTON'S SPACE[3]

We leave theology for the moment and consider how Newton arrived at the idea of infinite, homogeneous, three-dimensional, immovable and absolute space. The death-blow had, in fact, already been delivered to the Aristotelean system of the world by Copernicus' heliocentric system (1543). Kepler discovered the elliptic path of the planets (1609) and Newton discovered that the same force that causes heavy objects to fall downwards on earth is responsible for the paths of the moon and the planets (1687). This undermined Aristotle's theory that different laws of movement applied in the sublunar world than outside it. But that did not prove that space was—as Gassendi thought—absolute, immovable and infinite. Galileo had even stated that movement and immobility were relative terms. If an object was dropped from a tower it landed at the foot of the tower and if the same object was dropped from the crow's nest of a sailing ship it landed at the foot of the mast. But Newton declared that this relativity principle only applied in the kinematic sense: for spatial systems which were moving in a linear, uniform manner in relation to each other. When reference systems revolve in relation to each other, different dynamic laws apply. If the water in a revolving bucket is made to revolve, the water rises against the inside wall of the bucket. In this case one of the systems revolves

[2] Grant, 1981.
[3] Westfall, 1980.

and centrifugal forces are produced, while the other, absolute space, remains stationary and is therefore not subjected to any forces. In addition to absolute space, Newton also believed in absolute time.

Newton had influential critics, among them Leibnitz. Leibnitz declared, in a famous correspondence with Newton's representative Clarke, that space was only something relative, an order of coexistence of things, just as time was relative, an order of successive events. The tenor of the correspondence between Leibnitz and Clarke was mainly theological. Leibnitz opposed the theory that space was God or one of his attributes. But Leibnitz had no answer to Newton's dynamic argument.

In this way theology retreated from the field of space and Newton was victorious on physical grounds, a victory which for centuries would not be contested. But then two important new insights into physical space arose, which were to sound the knell of Newton's absolute space. The first insight was mathematical: the geometry of space; the second was physical: problems concerning the ether and the fields of force.

THE GEOMETRY OF SPACE

Newton saw his space, in agreement with Gassendi and his supporters, as infinite, boundless, immovable, homogeneous and three-dimensional. In this empty space particles of a given mass were moving according to the laws of mechanics, which were subject to Euclidean geometry. For Newton Euclidean geometry was literally the geometry of the earth, and as such a branch of mechanics.

Later, the perception grew that Euclidean geometry reflected the real world, but that other forms of geometry were conceivable, which might not be applicable to the real world, but to other—possible, hypothetical—worlds in which there are more than three dimensions or where space is curved and perhaps not even infinite. I mention only the German mathematician Riemann (1854), who demonstrated that so-called elliptic space could be finite, boundless and homogeneous at the same time.

HOW EMPTY IS SPACE?

Even in antiquity the ether was recognized, the *quinta essentia* which fills the space between the planets and between the fixed stars. Newton also fell back on this mysterious substance here and there in his Opticks (1704), and when Thomas Young demonstrated that light consisted of vibrations (1802), it had to be accepted that space was filled with ether which formed the medium for the vibrations of light. On another plane also, space was found to be less empty than had been assumed. Faraday (1791–1867) sprinkled iron filings on a sheet of paper and held a magnet under it. The iron filings arranged themselves into lines of force. Apparently space was not only a void filled with material objects, but it was also a *field of forces*. Space had structure. The Scottish physicist Maxwell, who combined electricity and magnetism into one system, attempted to define this structure (1873).

THE PRINCIPLE OF SPECIAL RELATIVITY

The study of asymmetries between electricity and magnetism led Einstein to the conclusion that physical laws always have the same validity independent of the reference system in which the researcher is making his measurements (1905; see Einstein, 1917). With this conclusion he finally laid to rest Newton's absolute space and the ether. There were two conditions: the reference systems had to move with constant velocity and in a rectilinear direction (as in Galileo's relativity principle), and the speed of light, which necessarily influences the measurements, had to be taken into consideration. In this way, time became included in every physical calculation. Relativistic physics doesn't think any more in terms of three-dimensional space but in a four-dimensional space-time continuum. In relation to spatial vision, the subject of this book, this relativity principle is not important. The speed of light is so great that it makes no difference whether one looks out of the window of a moving car or of one that is standing still. If the speed of light were 30 km per hour instead of 300,000 km per second[4], the relativity principle would have a great influence on how we see the world. A moving cyclist would appear much thinner than a stationary one and, at the same time, the cyclist would see the people on the pavement suddenly become much thinner as he rode away (Fig. 1.1).

THE PRINCIPLE OF GENERAL RELATIVITY

In Einstein's general theory of relativity, gravity, which is nothing more than a uniform acceleration, is included in the equivalence of physical reference systems (1915; see Einstein, 1917). This mathematical operation demanded that the structure of space should be positively curved in Riemann's sense, and thereby finite, although unbounded. In addition, distortions of space in the vicinity of celestial bodies had to be assumed. With the theory of general relativity, therefore, Newtonian space lost both its claim to infinity and its homogeneity. It soon became apparent that stellar systems are moving away from each other at great speed. Space is expanding, and had evidently been formed by a sort of explosion, the Big Bang. The theory of general relativity is indispensable to astronomy, but makes no difference to the world as we see it.

THE QUANTUM THEORY

Just as the theory of relativity is too big for human vision, microphysics, quantum mechanics, is too small. It is not important for our macroscopic behaviour in space, that energy is subdivided into units (quanta) and multiples of these (Planck, 1900). Even though there is tremendous unrest in the world of small things, and the fluctuations become greater as the area examined becomes smaller, we are completely unaware of it, because all the unrest is statistically levelled out in the world which lies open to our senses.

The theory of large things and the theory of small things are difficult to reconcile with each other. The wild fluctuations on the ultramicroscopic scale, as implied by the uncertainty principle of quantum mechanics, are irreconcilable with the sleek geometry of time-space which is the central principle of general relativity. The *string theory* is an attempt to solve this paradox[5]. In this book it is only

[4] Gamov, 1940.
[5] Greene, 1999.

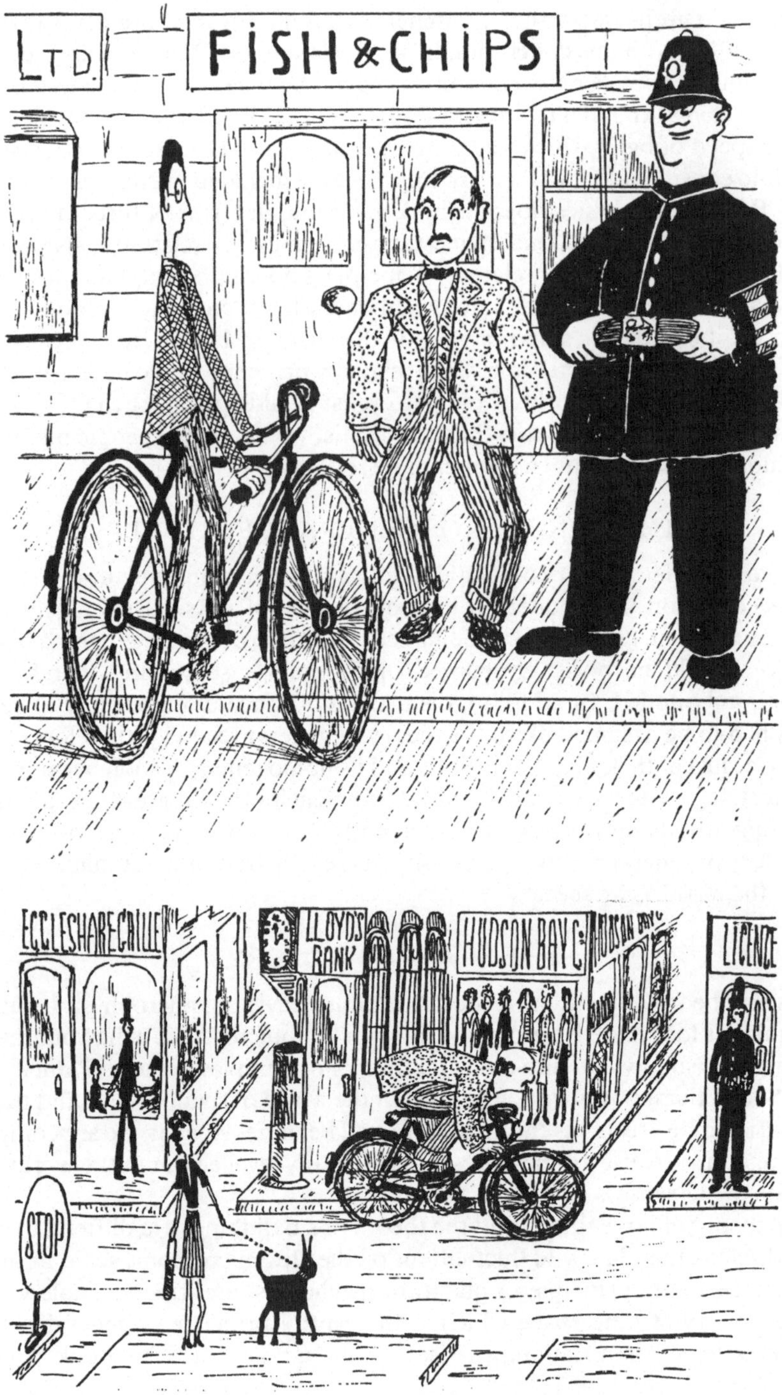

Fig. 1.1. If the speed of light were 30 Km/h the cyclist would look very thin from the pavement and the houses would appear very narrow to the cyclist (after Gamov, 1940).

important to know that the string theory operates in a world with ten or more dimensions. For the reader's peace of mind it may be said that even the string theory allots no more than three dimensions to macroscopic space; the other dimensions are, so to speak, the curled-up dimensions of a microworld. Even so, from Newton's absolute, homogeneous, infinite and three-dimensional world, the last attribute, the three-dimensionality, is now being called into question.

OBJECTIVE SPACE

The space, of which the history is sketched above, is distinguished as *real* space from geometrical spaces which are only a possibility, and also from any space which owes its existence solely to one or more—necessarily subjective—sensory qualities. Real space can also be called *physical* space, because it is not filled with visible, audible or tangible things, but with *measurable* objects. Because measurements can be verified or disproved by anybody, real space is also called *objective* space.

Classical physics has cut the connection between objective reality and the senses. That has led to enormous successes, to astonishing but completely dehumanised (without sensory information) knowledge. The separation of objective reality and the observer has, however, not been completely successful. Quantum mechanics is based once more on two corner-stones: the reality and the observer. In this case it is not the painting of reality in the colours of the human senses, but the alteration of reality by the action of a human measuring instrument.

2. Perceptual Space

HISTORICAL NOTES

In the previous chapter the objective features of space have been characterized; the question now arises how the spatial characteristics of things are *perceived*. To acquaint the reader with divergent theories, I introduce three founders of epistemology: Locke, Berkeley and Kant.

LOCKE: PRIMARY AND SECONDARY FEATURES

The explosive growth of physics during the scientific revolution is due to exclusive attention for the spatial, quantitative aspects of nature, associated with neglect of the sensory information. Galileo said that the book of nature was written in mathematical language. Scents, sounds and tastes were solely human experiences. Descartes, one of the most prominent theorists of mechanistic physics, made a rigid distinction between spatial magnitude, the *extensio*, and the *cogitatio*, thinking and feeling, including the special senses.

With his mechanics of the heavens, expounded in the *Principia*, Newton was able to give the final touch to the mechanistic vision of the world. In his other book, the *Opticks* (1704), however, he could not avoid to discuss the mental sensation of colour. In his research into the prismatic colour spectrum he managed to keep physics and psychology strictly separate. He was intensely interested in the refraction of light, but also in the phenomenology of sensations of colour. Rays of light, he stated, are distinguishable by their physical properties, such as the size of the light particles, but *have no colour of their own*. It is only when they stimulate the retina that colour arises in the psyche.

Locke, the English philosopher, shared his friend Newton's opinion. The difference between the spatial and the sensory has, thanks to Locke, become defined as the difference between *primary and secondary qualities*. The primary qualities included, according to Locke, spatial extent and form, number, movement and impenetrability. He called colour, scent, palpability and sound secondary qualities. In his book on the theory of knowledge, his *Essay Concerning Human Understanding* (1690), he stated that our knowledge of the primary qualities corresponds with the things themselves, whereas our understanding of the secondary qualities of things has no resemblance to their objective characteristics.

BERKELEY

The theory of primary and secondary qualities did not remain unchallenged. There are two alternatives: either colour is as objective as space, or space is as subjective as colour. The first alternative is called 'naïve realism,' the second 'idealism.' The English philosopher Berkeley was an idealist. He said in his *Principles of Human Knowledge* (1710) that form and colour have the same status: that of sensory phenomena. The form in which an object is observed is dependent on the observer. A horse in the distance is small and a horse nearby is big; a wheel is seen as circular or elliptical according to the position of the observer. Our sense of space is the sense of space of the genus Mankind, and as such is subjective: a mite, according to Berkeley, would not be able to exist if it did not have a completely different sense of space, adjusted to shorter distances and different spatial information. Berkeley found objective space absurd. Space is *phenomenal*, defined by the spatial impressions which we receive; he denied the objective existence of matter. *Esse est percipi*: all that exists is what is perceived. Berkeley is a consistent spiritualist. God's creation consists of nothing more than perceiving spirits and perceived sensations (ideas). Berkeley didn't go so far as to say that the world disappeared when one closed one's eyes: the world always remained in God's sensorium. God's spirit is the all-embracing spirit. Because all knowledge is built up from sensory impressions, and abstract ideas like the concept of substance are rejected, Berkeley is also a consistent empiricist. His revolutionary theory of knowledge was inspired by his antirevolutionary Christian conviction, unsympathetic to materialists, atheists and free-thinkers.

Berkeley's theory later became popular in secularised form, particularly among psychologists and philosophers, as *phenomenalism*. Phenomenalism forms a poor basis for the natural sciences. Theoretical chemistry cannot be built on scents and colours, and without abstractions one cannot get far with Newton's gravitation law.

KANT

Even so, it was a Newtonian who made the 'subjectivity' (or rather: the non-objectivity) of space in his *Kritik der reinen Vernunft* (1781) a corner-stone of his philosophical system. Kant asked himself the question, what is the reason for the irrefutable validity of Euclid's axioms and Newton's mechanistic laws? His answer: space is an 'a-priori intuition,' a classification scheme for the human intellect into which knowledge must organize itself. Space (and time also) does not form, for Kant, part of the objective reality but is a product of 'pure' (aprioristic) human reason. Kant does not elaborate on what remains of nature if all the contributions of human reason are removed. The 'thing-in-itself' is the source of all experience but is not directly accessible to knowledge.

One might suppose that Kant, with his theory, had eliminated the distinction between primary and secondary qualities, but that is far from being the case. The sensory, such as colour, is in Kant's view immeasurable and, on account of its individual subjectivity, fortuitous. On the other hand, the ideality of space is 'transcendental,' a supra-individual requirement of human knowledge. Kantian space, although 'de-objectified' in the epistemological sense, remained in practice the 'objective' space of the physicists and not the phenomenal space of the psychologists and their great leader, Berkeley. Kant called his own idealism 'critical,' in order to distinguish it from the (in his opinion) 'sentimental' idealism of Berkeley.

The ideas of the Enlightenment culminated in the philosophy of Kant. His influence was unprecedented. Together with the classical writers in Weimar, he made a deep impression on German spiritual life. Preachers' sons and theology students, already disturbed by the Enlightenment, adopted Kant's doctrine. They were more familiar with Plato, Goethe and the Gospels than with empirical natural science. The first thing they did was throw the 'thing-in-itself' overboard. Without the ballast of experience, thought could rise to speculative heights where 'thinking thinks itself.'

The rapid advance of the natural sciences put an end to this sort of idealism. Materialism won the sympathy of many. As, however, materialism did not form a sufficient basis for the sensory sciences with their mental phenomena, others returned to Locke's and Kant's original theories. Hermann von Helmholtz, great practitioner of the sensory sciences and also mathematician and physicist, had in his theory of colour vision (based on Thomas Young) stated that it depends on the properties of the eye which 'signals' we use to interpret reality. As the retina has three sorts of receptors, our collection of colours is threefold. The retina is the 'creator of colour.' Some philosophers and investigators of the special senses tried to demonstrate that the senses which register space were, in the same way, 'creators of space.' They hoped in this way to lay a scientific basis for Kant's subjectivism, against Kant's intentions, who had specifically stated that space is not an empirical term.

All these attempts stranded. Some neo-Kantians tried to interpret space through feelings experienced in muscles and joints, by means of which we learn the difference between above and below, before and behind and left and right. The physiologist Cyon used the directional feelings produced by the three semicircular canals of the organ of equilibrium. His article (1901) had the characteristic title *The physiological basis of Euclid's geometry. A solution of the space problem.* Unhappily the semicircular canals were already expressed in spatial terms. The argument was thus begging the question, it was a *petitio principii.*

We have now heard three philosophers who, in spite of all their brain-racking, were not able to formulate an idea of space which is acceptable to us.

Locke represented the position of the new natural science from Galileo to Newton. He made two mistakes. In the first place, we don't observe space 'as it is.' Our observation is, as far as the visual observation is concerned, dependent on our own viewpoint and the properties of the eye. In the second place, it is a scientistic error to think that sounds (mental sensatione which can be scientifically reduced to vibrations in the air), are less real than vibrations in the air.

Berkeley rejected the scientism of his time and argued that all our knowledge was sensory. He was an 'immaterialist,' who denied the objective existence of things. It was an extreme position which could not last. It was irreconcilable with the natural science which was rapidly developing, and was also contrary to the daily experience of ordinary people.

Kant tried to explain the strict validity of natural laws by the statement that 'space' was a fundamental category of the human spirit. This standpoint was not tenable either. As explained in Chapter 1, an objective physical space exists which is certainly not the product of the human spirit. In addition, Kant's theory was highly anthropocentric and no reference was made to what spatial behaviour means in the animal world.

It seems important to us, modern people, to define space in such a way that the definition applies for physics (Chapter 1), for biology and for the human spirit.

BIOLOGICAL ASPECTS OF SPATIAL LOCALISATION

Organisms have special senses that collect information which is of importance for their lives, and pass it on to their motor apparatus, so that the organism can react adequately to the information.

This takes place in even the most primitive animals. Unicellular organisms can have a 'receptor' in their cell wall which registers a gradient in the concentration of a given fluid in their environment, and which sends this stimulus on to another part of the cell wall, where there is a whiplash which moves the cell in the direction of the chemical substance or in the other direction, as required.

In higher animals the 'receptors' are highly specialized cells which react sensitively to physical or chemical changes in their environment and pass on their stimulated condition via a nerve fibre. Examples of such receptors are the rods and cones in the retina and the hair-cells in the labyrinth. The receptors are the essential part of the sensory organs, in this case of the eye and the organ of equilibrium. We can speak of a *sensory system* when the spatial information is obtained from many scattered receptors. Thus mechanoreceptors in the skin, muscles and joints form a complicated system that we call 'proprioceptive,' in so far as it registers stimuli that lead to correction of the position of the body, and more broadly speaking 'sense of touch,' when objects in the outside world are the cause of the stimulation.

When sensory stimuli contain spatial information, movement usually occurs, a *sensorimotor reaction*. Thus a falling cat positions itself while falling with the help of stimuli from its organ of equilibrium. A deer turns its head when it hears something rustle in the wood. A fly flies away when it sees an approaching hand. These are all sensorimotor processes that can be described in biological terms. The spatial localization of animals often differs greatly from that of humans. While we follow a trail with the help of visible footprints, a dog follows the same trail with his nose. Snakes possess an organ which is sensitive to warmth, by means of which they localise their prey. Bats transmit ultrasonic vibrations reflected by insects; the bat's ears localise the insect.

PSYCHOLOGICAL ASPECTS OF SPATIAL LOCALISATION

ANIMALS AND PSYCHOLOGY

Is there any point in asking how it feels to be a bat?[1] For practical reasons we must answer this question in the negative. It is almost impossible to enter into the inner world of another human being, let alone of a bat. The question is, whether such a query is theoretically justified: has a bat an inner world of feelings or not? There

[1] Nagel, 1974.

are two extreme opinions on this question, both associated with illustrious names. *Descartes* considered animals to be 'automatons' without feelings. He only allowed feelings and thought to human beings. A pregnant dog was kicked out of the room by Malebranche, a younger follower of Descartes[2]. When the animal began to yelp pitifully, he said to his guests: 'it's only a machine.'

Leibnitz, who was opposed to Descartes' materialism, thought that even the humblest animals had a soul and *petites perceptions*. Most modern people take a middle course. If a cat screams when someone steps on his tail, that is thought to be an expression of pain, and when he butts you with his head, that is taken to be an expression of affection. But the expressive movements of a fly? If they exist, we cannot recognize them. Which doesn't mean to say that flies are 'machines,' but only that we allow animals an inner life on the grounds of recognizable behaviour.

PSYCHOLOGICAL DESCRIPTION OF THE HUMAN BEING

For human beings it is possible to give, in addition to a biological description of spatial behaviour, a *psychological* description. The space we experience exists thanks to our senses. Phenomenal, perceptual space is a *mental* space with the perceiving self in the centre, a space *that exists in our consciousness and is therefore the domain of psychology.* Motor action also takes place in the phenomenal space. The self directs its eyes towards an object, turns its head, grasps with its hands. These movements often have a quality that does not appear in biological descriptions: they are purposeful, intentional.

But the world that is perceptible through the senses does not only belong to our private internal domain; we see a cyclist riding on the other side of the street and we don't think for a moment that the cyclist is only part of our internal life. The world we experience with our senses is subjectively conditioned, but not subjective. Nevertheless, it is good to realize that we see the cyclist in our personal (although 're-objectivated'), mentally constructed—and coloured—world, not just as a scientific object, localized in the coordinates of physical space, reflecting light rays of a given wavelength.

Perceptual space is thus built on two foundations: objective space on the one hand and the mental perception and action of the observer on the other. The mental component consists of heterogeneous information, deriving from our eyes and ears, our organs of equilibrium and of touch, and our motor receptors. All these data from the senses are not automatically correlated with each other. If we look at a railway line we see the rails in the distance getting steadily closer to each other, but if we feel the distance between the rails with our arms it appears that it is the same everywhere. This is just one example, but there are innumerable situations in which the spatial particulars supplied by the various senses are not in agreement.

REAL SPACE AS PROOF STATION FOR PHENOMENAL SPACE

The objective space described in Chapter 1, is the space of physics. It is also the real space which forms the indispensable proof station in which all sensory information

[2] van Hoorn, 1972.

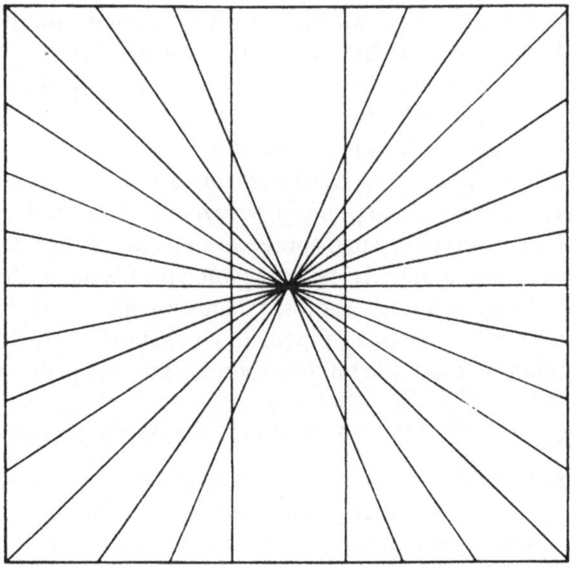

Fig. 2.1. An optical illusion: the vertical lines appear to be bent, but they are straight.

is assessed and checked as to its verity. The mensuration of physical space gives the final answer, as in the optical illusion in Figure 2.1, where the ruler proves that the left and right vertical lines are not curved, although our visual perception makes us believe that they are.

THE PLACE OF BIOLOGY AND PSYCHOLOGY IN A PLURALISTIC WORLD

The biological and the psychological approaches are complementary. We have, as already stated, absolutely no reason to deny animals a psyche, but, for the analysis of their sensations and intentions, we have to rely on the objective study of their behaviour. With human beings, we can enquire into the content of their spatial sensations and intentions. These are sometimes so subtle that they cannot be recognized in the spatial behaviour of the subject but, on the other hand, a lot of spatial information does not penetrate into consciousness, so that objective study of spatial behaviour has a function in humans also.

There is unmistakably a *pluralistic* hierarchy[3] in our real world: the basis is *matter,* which is the subject of physics. Above matter comes *life*, which has different laws from 'dead' matter. Nevertheless, the material, world is the foundation of life. Biologists occupy themselves with life. Above life comes the *mind*, the domain of psychologists. With the arrival of the mental, the subjective, something quite new appears on the world stage, with quite different laws from those of life. The laws of the mind still have their foundation in the laws of biology, but not all laws which

[3] Hartmann, 1947.

apply to the material and the biological world are still applicable to the mental domain. Thus feelings are not susceptible to the exact measurements that exist in the area of physics. Furthermore, the mind—although dependent on the existence of the individual—can transcend his material and biological limits. I have already stated that subjective visual space is a mental space. The same is true for subjective acoustic space. The fourth element in the structure of our real world is *culture*. Culture is founded on the individual minds, but obeys its own laws. It is striking that the most typical feature of the individual mind, the subjectivity, has been lost in the culture.

Many attempts to simplify the plurality of this image of the world have been made. A first step is 'dualism,' the sharp distinction between matter and soul which goes back to René Descartes. In this theory the independent existence of life is thrown overboard and culture is degraded to psychologism. A still further simplification is 'monism,' the reduction of existence to one domain. Berkeley was the representative of psychic monism. The present triumphal march of the natural sciences has caused materialistic monism to have the most adherents.

In this study on spatial vision the cultural element is not taken into consideration. But the relationship between biology and psychology will continually demand our attention. As biology is ontologically more fundamental than psychology, the biological approach to the special senses has in theory precedence. But psychology produces such a wealth of subjective information that it has an important place in this book.

THE AREA BETWEEN PERCEPTION AND ACTION

Between the perception of phenomenal space and possible resulting action (both subjects of psychological investigation) there is a broad area which is not available to psychology, but on physical examination reveals a large number of important facts. This is the domain of anatomy and physiology. These sciences begin with the structure and function of the receptor organs and end with the structure and function of the effector systems (the eye muscles, mechanism of hand and foot movements, etc.). The largest place in objective sensory science is occupied by neurophysiology, a discipline which has recently produced remarkable insights but which is still in its infancy.

3. Non-Visual Spatial Perception

INTRODUCTION

THE ORGAN OF EQUILIBRIUM

The organs of equilibrium (labyrinth, vestibule), situated in mammals in the petrous bone, are extremely important for non-visual spatial perception. The labyrinth is a double organ, in the first place consisting of the *utriculus* and the *sacculus.* These contain lumps of calcium carbonate, the so-called otoliths, which by their weight can exert pressure on receptor cells. The organs register the direction of gravity and other linear accelerations. In the second place, the three *semicircular canals*, which are at right angles to each other (Fig. 3.1) and are filled with fluid, the endolymph. When the head is turned a flow originates in the endolymph, giving rise to stimulation of the receptors in the dilated end of each canal, the so-called ampulla. In this way the canals register the turning of the head in the three

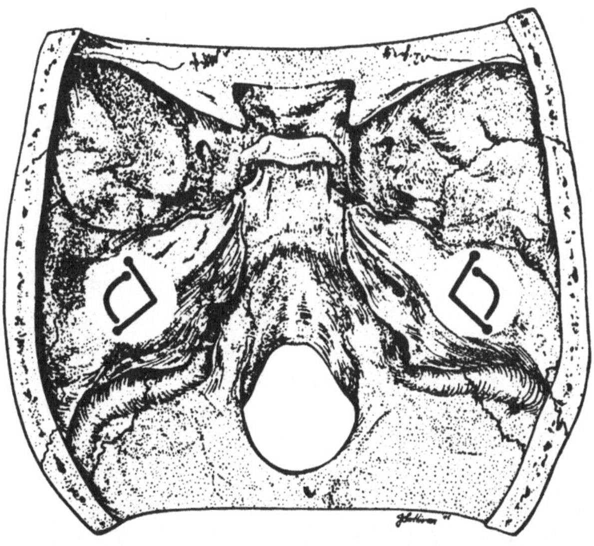

Fig. 3.1. Diagram of the position of the semicircular canals and their ampullae in the skull (Cogan, 1948).

dimensions of objective space. In the central nervous system the nerve fibres arising from the labyrinth enter the vestibular nuclei, which are closely connected with the centres from which movements are controlled: the motor centres in the spinal cord, the cerebrum and the cerebellum. There is a particularly close relationship between the organ of equilibrium and the motor centres for eye movements. This will be considered in Chapter 5.

KINAESTHESIS AND TOUCH

The non-visual perception of movement and of the direction of gravity is called 'proprioception.' Not only the labyrinths are responsible for this sense, but also the 'kinaesthetic' mechanoreceptors in the skin, muscles and joints. When an aeroplane accelerates for the take-off, we feel the pressure of the seat against our backs. When we slip we feel changes in the tension and position of our bodies, resulting in a movement which restores our balance.

Touch, in the wider conception of kinaesthesia, is, after vision, the most important aid to the exploration of space. A touch sensation does not only arise from stimulation of pressure-sensitive receptors in the skin. Information from position-sensitive receptors in the joints and tension-sensitive receptors in the muscles are also indispensable for good tactile perception.

The space which we perceive with the senses of touch (and balance) has much in common with objective space, although it is naturally very restricted. There are three equal dimensions at right angles to each other: the vertical, lateral and antero-posterior co-ordinates. In view of the biological importance of gravity and the bilateral symmetry of our bodies, these are the most natural co-ordinates.

TOUCH AND VISION IN HISTORICAL PERSPECTIVE[1]

In anticipation of the following chapters, we may already say that visual space corresponds much less well with objective space than tactile space. The depth co-ordinate in visual space has a distinctive characteristic: parallel lines appear to converge at a distance and circles may resemble ellipses. Spatial vision is clearly more susceptible to illusions than touch. Since time immemorial it has been known that the eyes can easily be deceived. If you want to be sure if a long-lost friend is suddenly standing in front of you in the flesh, you only have to stretch out your arms: touch is the guarantee for reality!

No one can deny that the visual experience of space is infinitely richer than the tactile experience. But it is still possible that the visual experience is too uncertain and deceptive to be adequate without touch. This is the main problem which confronted sensory psychology in its early days (Fig. 3.2). The discussion received a strong impulse when William Molyneux, a leading Irish lawyer, politician and practitioner of optics, asked Locke a famous question: '*Suppose a man born blind, and now adult, and taught by his touch to distinguish between a cube and a sphere. Suppose then the blind man to be made to see: quaere, whether by his sight, before he touched them, he could now distinguish and tell which is the globe, which the cube?*'

[1] Pastore, 1971; Degenaar, 1996.

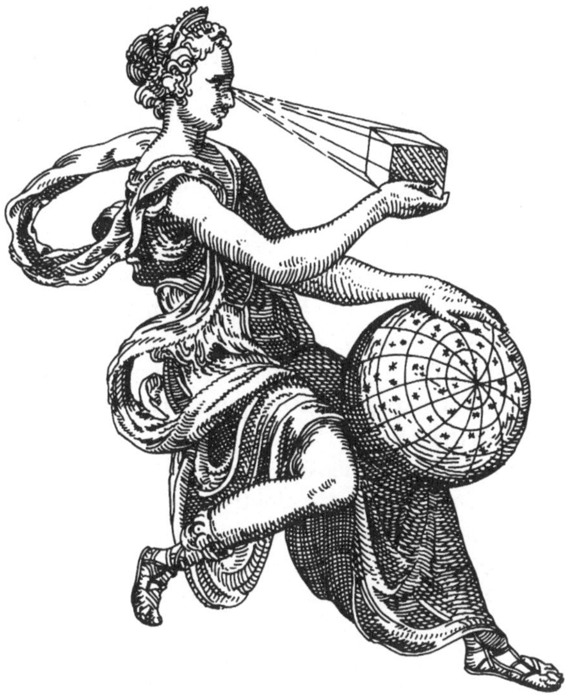

Fig. 3.2. Touch and vision. From Jamnizer, *Perspectiva corporum regularium* (1568).

To which the acute and judicious proposer answers: '*Not. For though he has obtained the experience of how a globe, how a cube affects his touch, yet he has not yet obtained the experience that what affects his touch so or so must affect his sight so or so.*' Locke continues: '*I agree with this thinking gentleman, whom I am proud to call my friend.*'

Locke, already mentioned in connection with primary and secondary qualities, was also the philosopher of empirism, the theory that all knowledge arises from experience and that inborn knowledge does not exist. It is understandable that the empirist Locke agrees with Molyneux: the visual impressions of the sphere and the cube fall on a *tabula rasa*, a blank tablet. Before the cube and the sphere can be recognized and named, an association must be made by experience between the tactile and the visual impressions. There are no 'innate ideas' which equate the terminologies of touch and vision.

Thirty years later Molyneux's empiristic ideas seemed to be confirmed. In 1728 the famous ophthalmologist William Cheselden wrote in the Philosophical Transactions: *An Account of some Observations made by a young Gentleman, who was born blind, or lost his Sight so early, that he had no Remembrance of ever having seen, and was couch'd between 13 and 14 Years of Age.* The result of the cataract stab seemed at first to be disappointing: '*When he first saw, he was so far from making any Judgements about Distances, that he thought all Objects whatever touch'd his Eyes (as he express'd it) as what he felt, did his skin. He knew not the Shape of anything, nor any one Thing from another, however different in Shape, or in Magnitude: but on being told what Things were, whose Form he before knew from feeling, he would carefully observe, that he might know them again.'* Later he began to discover shapes, also in pictures, but he was amazed to find that painted shapes felt flat. Apparently he derived experiences of depth from tactile memories and not from the visual image itself. But all's well that ends well: *'A Year after first seeing, being carried on Epsom Downs, and observing a large Prospect, he was exceedingly delighted with it, and call'd it a new Kind of Seeing.'*

The empirists considered this case history to be decisive proof of their own theory. Voltaire described the case in his much read *Elémens de la philosophie de Newton* (1738) and the encyclopedist Diderot gave an extensive analysis of Cheselden's report in his *Lettre sur les aveugles, á l'usage de ceux qui voient* (1751). Another encyclopedist, the naturalist Buffon (1707–1788), was also convinced of the precedence of tactile sensations over our experience of space. He called the sense of touch the 'sens géométrique.' From the point of view of physics, that was an attractive idea. It is not surprising that geometry uses measures associated with touch, such as foot and ell. In comparison, the visual world is geometrically very primitive and, in Buffon's view, only two-dimensional! Vision can learn a lot from touch. In Buffon's own words: 'Before touch teaches children the true position of things and their own bodies, they see everything upside down. A second defect in their vision at this stage is that they see things double, because each eye forms its own image. Only the experience of touch can correct this fault, and it does this so well that we finally believe that we see things single and right side up. We ascribe this impression to vision, but in fact it derives from touch.'

NATIVISM AND EMPIRISM

Viewed from the perspective of our present knowledge, no proof at all can be based on a case like Cheselden's. The renowned patient (and every similar one in later centuries) had missed the chance, because of his lengthy spell of blindness, to learn to see at the right time and therefore needed much time to catch up on his visual retardation. This is merely a medico-physiological question, with no possible consequences for the epistemology. I shall return to this in more detail in the chapter on squint.

In the meantime the pendulum which had swung too far to the side of empirism had begun to return to the centre. Kant reinstated the *a priori* and declared that the intuition of space preceded every other experience. A sharp blow was dealt to empirism when Wheatstone discovered the stereoscopic perception of depth in 1838. This robbed the empiricists of their principal argument: that in-depth vision was dependent on the sense of touch. Other scientific observations were also brought into alignment against empirism. For instance, examination of babies showed that indications of spatial vision were present before significant tactile experience had been gained. These observations refuted empirism and supported the opposite point of view, 'nativism.'

The controversy between empirists and nativists continued for a long time in the field of the special senses, as a grim battle between rival sects. The German physiologist Hering (1834–1894) was a convinced nativist, on the grounds of his study of binocular vision. Helmholtz (1821–1894), who worked largely in the same field, remained an empiricist. The last chapter of his famous Handbook is a plea for the concept that spatial vision is dependent on experience and associations.

Now we no longer need to take sides in this struggle which lasted well into the twentieth century. The chapter on squint and amblyopia will make it clear that inborn ability and experience go hand in hand. The sense of sight has much to learn in the course of the development of the young organism, but in this process it is dominant and an autodidact, and does not need the sense of touch as teacher. Man is an optical animal. The optic nerves contain more nerve fibres than those reaching the cerebral cortex from all other sensory systems together. The visual system also occupies more space in the cerebral cortex than any other sensory system. We can therefore have an easy conscience when we direct our attention in Part II of this book to the study of spatial vision, as a separate entity, without initially considering its relationship with the sense of touch.

Part II: The Visual Perception of Space

4. Some Basic Facts about the Visual System

THE EYE AND THE OCULAR MUSCLES

THE OPTICS OF THE EYE

A horizontal section through the eyeball is shown in Figure 4.1. Few of the details need to be considered in this book. The eye is an optical system with two lenses. The front of the cornea is the surface with the greatest refractive power. The lens itself has less refractive power, but this is variable because the thickness of the lens can change. Parallel rays falling straight into the eye are focussed onto the centre of the *fovea*, the centre of the retina. When the lens is made thicker (accommodation, Fig. 4.2), a sharp image of near objects is obtained. With age the ability to accommodate

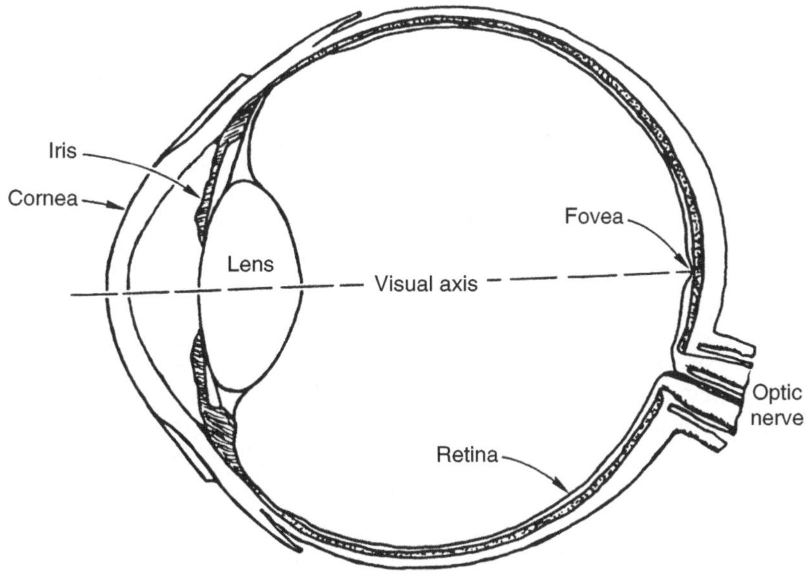

Fig. 4.1. Cross-sectional diagram of the human eye (Cornsweet, 1970).

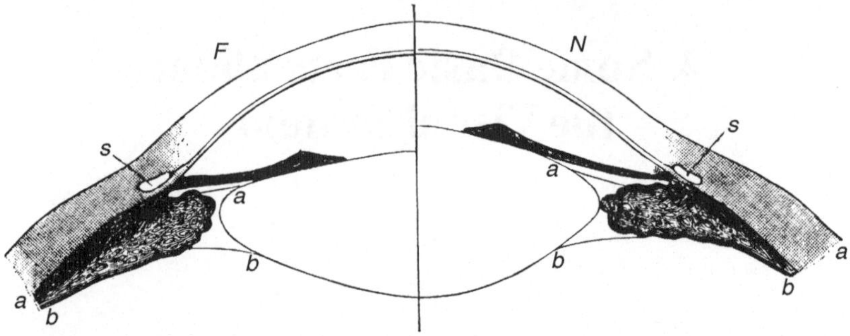

Fig. 4.2. Accommodation. Contraction of a circular muscle round the lens makes the lens thicker (Helmholtz, 1866).

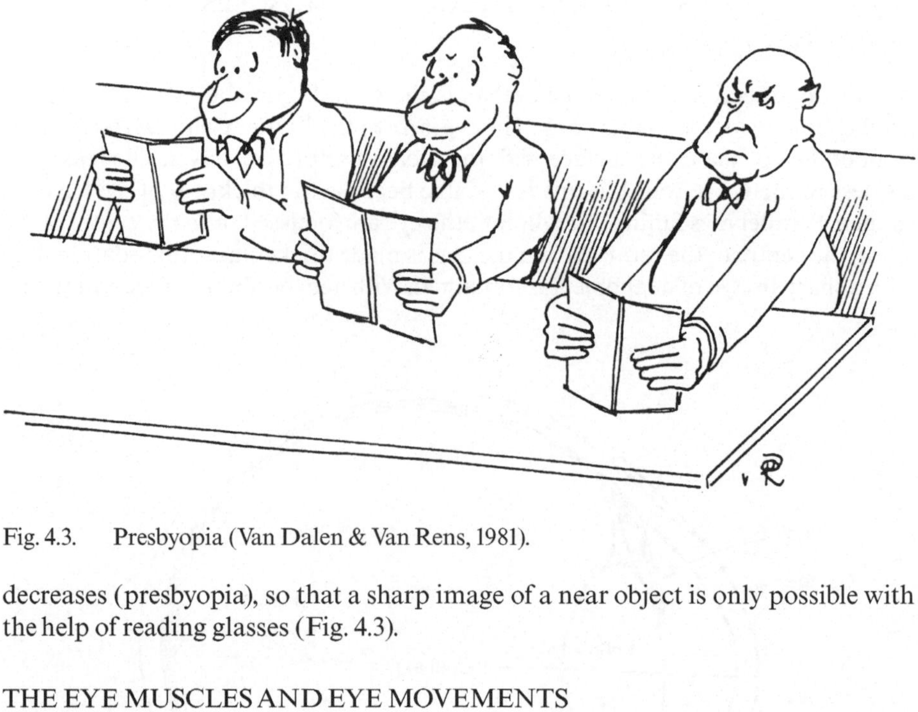

Fig. 4.3. Presbyopia (Van Dalen & Van Rens, 1981).

decreases (presbyopia), so that a sharp image of a near object is only possible with the help of reading glasses (Fig. 4.3).

THE EYE MUSCLES AND EYE MOVEMENTS

Each eye has six external eye muscles, four straight and two oblique (Fig. 4.4). The inner and outer muscles turn the eye round a vertical axis. The other muscles all turn the eye in both a vertical, a horizontal and a torsional direction. This complicated situation need not worry us (unless one of the muscles becomes paralysed). In normal life the muscles work together in such a way that two sorts of movements are possible: simple horizontal and vertical movements (and combinations of these) and pure torsional movements (round the antero-posterior 'sagittal' axis).

The *control* of these eye movements takes place in the brain stem and the cerebellum. The machinery is there which, in numerous nuclei and nerve fibre

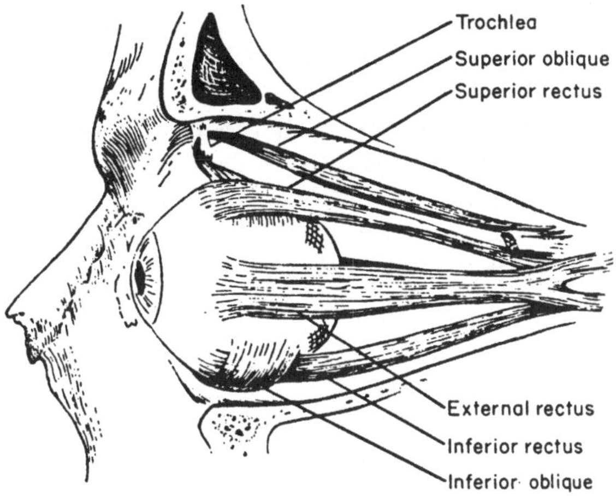

Fig. 4.4. Origins and insertions of the extraocular muscles (Cogan, 1948).

connections, is responsible for the simultaneous rapid jerks and slower following movements of the two eyes, and also for the slow movements in opposite directions. Much is known about the subcortical structures and their functions. The details are beyond the scope of this book, but a few principles will be considered in the following chapters.

Some knowledge of the *nomenclature* of the eye movements is necessary for the reader of this book. I shall restrict myself to the horizontal and torsional movements. When only one eye is being considered, one speaks of *ductions.* Movements of the two eyes in the same direction (conjugated movements) are called *versions*, movements in opposite directions (disjunctive movements) are *vergences.* Thus, apart from vertical movements, we speak of:

1. Adduction (inwards), abduction (outwards); incycloduction, excycloduction (upper pole of the cornea moves inwards/outwards);
2. Dextroversion, sinistroversion; dextrocycloversion, sinistrocycloversion;
3. Convergence, divergence; incyclovergence, excyclovergence.

THE RETINA

From Greek antiquity to the Renaissance people always thought that the organ of vision was the lens. The retina was known to exist as a thin membrane in which (on account of the course of the blood vessels) a fishing-net could be seen, but there was no reason to pay further attention to it.

Interest was awakened when the Basle anatomist Felix Platter (1536–1614) was persuaded that the lens was an *optic* element of the eye and localised the light sensibility at the back of the eye. The same idea had also been entertained by Vesalius. He thought that the place where the optic nerve leaves the eye was the light-sensitive spot. But Platter went further. He called the retina the 'retiform nerve' and declared that this was the light-sensitive structure. He saw the lens as a sort of internal spectacle glass through which the eye looked at the outside world. He did not understand the passage of light rays in the eye, but the idea that the retina consisted of light-sensitive nervous tissue was new and extremely important.

Johannes Kepler (1571–1630) was the first to understand the path of light rays in the eye. In about 1600 he discovered that the image of the outside world was projected upside down on the retina. People would not believe this at first, but by dissecting the back of a cow's eye down to the transparent retina, people were able to see the inverted image with their own eyes. Descartes made a nice illustration of this experiment (Fig. 4.5).

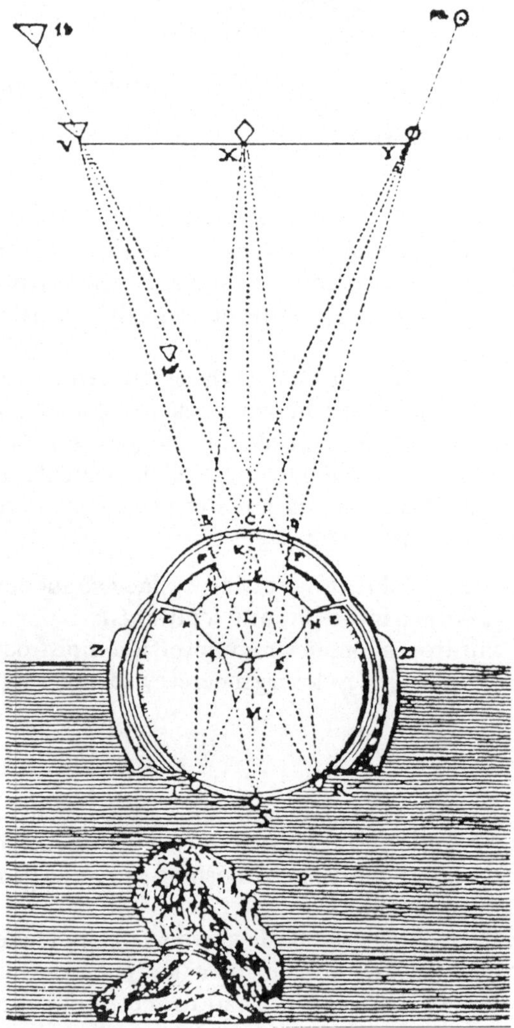

Fig. 4.5. The inverted image made visible. The posterior layers of the eye have been partly removed (Descartes, *Dioptrique*, [1637]).

The structure of this thin membrane was a problem for a long time. Since Schulze's study in 1863 (Fig. 4.6), nine layers have been distinguished in the retina. Thanks to the electron microscope many details have now become visible (Fig. 4.7). Two sorts of receptors, the rods and the cones, are found in the posterior layers, 7–9, of the retina. The cones are responsible for colour vision and the rods for vision in poor light. The fovea centralis, which consists of closely packed cones only, is a localized thinning of the retina. This has been produced by pushing the many other elements which lie between the cones and the nerves to one side (Fig. 4.8). Each foveal cone has its own connection with the central nervous system; this explains the high resolving power of the fovea centralis. In horizontal section (Fig. 4.9) the retina contains light-sensitive receptors up to 70 degrees on the temporal side and up to more than 90 degrees on the nasal side. The visual field therefore extends further on the temporal side than on the nasal side. The upper and lower limits of the visual field are a little closer to the centre.

Between the receptors and the nerve fibres of the optic nerve (Fig. 4.7) there lies, in layers 6 to 3, a complicated network of nerve fibres and nerve cells. On the inner

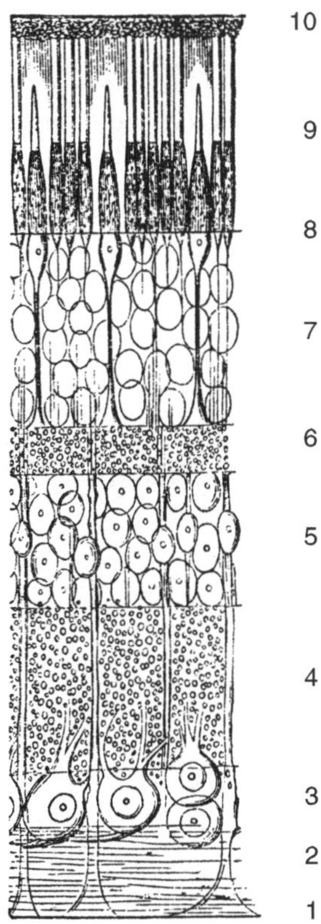

Fig. 4.6. Section of the retina (Schulze, 1863). Layer 2 (on the inside) contains the nerve fibres of the optic nerve, layer 9 the receptors.

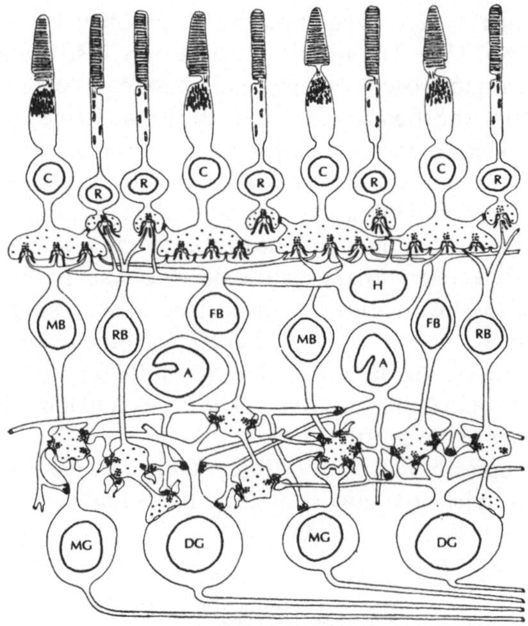

Fig. 4.7. Neural connections in the retina (Dowling, 1987). Cones (C) and rods (R) are connected directly and via horizontal cells (H). Some bipolars (MB) connect one cone with one ganglion cell (MG); others (FB, RB) transmit impulses from more than one receptor to larger ganglion cells (DG). The amacrine cells (A) make horizontal connections on the inner side of the outer plexiform layer.

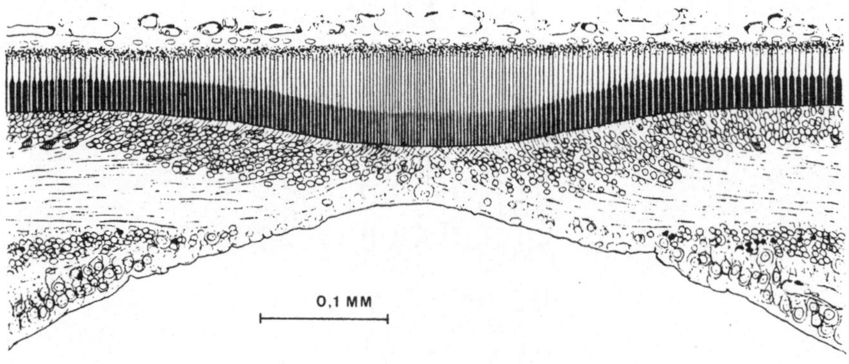

Fig. 4.8. Section of the fovea centralis (Polyak, 1948). The cones are elongated. Only at the extreme periphery of the preparation a few rods can be seen.

side of the retina the cell bodies (ganglion cells) are found, whose extensions form the fibres of the optic nerve. These fibres leave the eye at the optic disc and run for a short distance through the orbit and under the base of the brain, and then enter into the cerebrum.

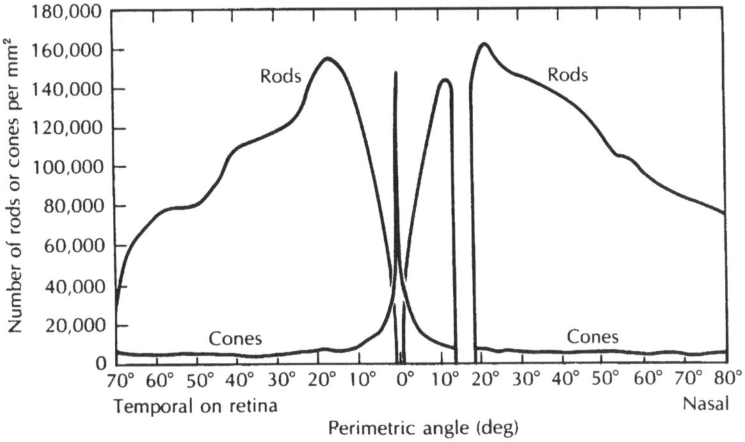

Fig. 4.9. Distribution of rods and cones in the retina. Counted in the horizontal meridian by Østerberg (1935).

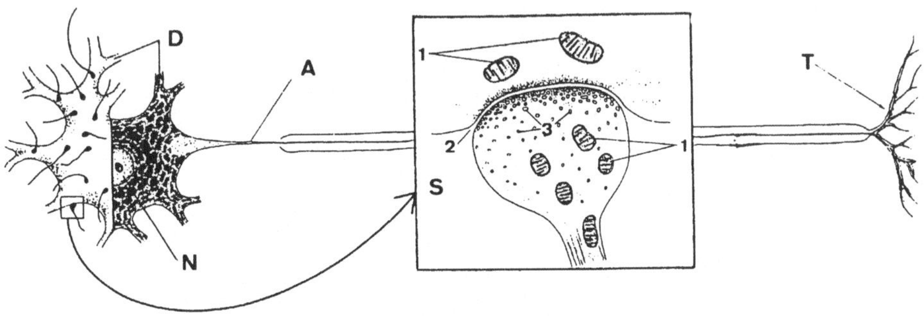

Fig. 4.10. Diagram of a nerve cell (after Bargmann, 1977). The outside of the cell body is seen on the left, a section on the right. (A) Axon; (D) dendrite; (N) nucleus; (S) synapse; (T) terminal arborisation. Extensions of other cells form synapses with dendrites and the cell body. In the centre of the diagram an enlarged synapse is shown. (1) Mitochondria; (2) synaptic cleft; (3) vesicles containing a substance which brings about the chemical transmission of the stimulus.

Figure 4.10 shows the basic structure of a nerve cell. This consists of a cell body, a dendrite and an axon. The dendrite consists of tree-like branches with which stimuli from adjacent cells are received. The axon, which may be extremely long, has branches at the end with which stimuli are passed to the other nerve cells, muscles and other organs. Nerve cells have many points of contact, the so-called synapses. The stimulated condition of a nerve cell is accompanied by electrical activity, but the stimuli are passed from one cell to another by chemical means.

THE VISUAL PATHWAYS[1]

When the fibres from the retina enter the brain they form synapses with numerous groups of cells ('nuclei'), which transport the information along various pathways and process it. Summary knowledge of the anatomy of the brain is necessary for the basic understanding of these visual pathways. Figure 4.11 shows a (half)lateral view of the brain. The brain stem can be seen with, above it, the cerebellum, which coordinates motor activity but is not considered in this book. Above this, the convoluted cerebral cortex is seen. The cortex consists of two hemispheres, which are each subdivided into four lobes: frontal, temporal, parietal and occipital. A small part of the occipital lobe is taken up by the striate area, the primary visual centre. Figure 4.12 shows schematically a horizontal section through the eyes and the fibre system leaving the retina and entering the brain at the point CGL (lateral geniculate body). A section of the brain stem is seen in the middle. In the section of the occipital lobe the visual fibres can be seen, running to the striate area (AS).

The *optic nerves* (*NO*) transport stimuli from the receptors to the brain. There are many millions of receptors in the retina, but the optic nerve contains not more than a million fibres. In the periphery of the retina many receptors (especially rods) are connected to the optic nerve by one fibre.

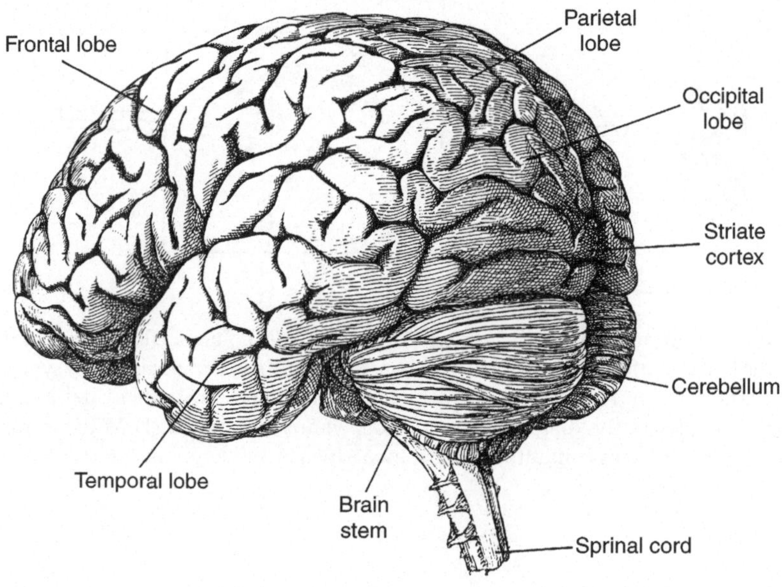

Fig. 4.11. Half-lateral view of the human brain, with the frontal, temporal, parietal and occipital lobes. The area striata, cerebellum, brainstem and spinal cord are also shown (after Hubel, 1988).

[1] Hubel, 1988; Fischer and Boch, 1991; Zeki, 1993.

In the *optic chiasma* the optic nerves cross each other in an X-shaped structure. Only the fibres from the nasal halves of the retinas cross, the fibres from the temporal halves go straight on (semidecussation, Fig. 4.12).

The *optic tracts* are the continuation of the optic nerves into the base of the brain at the level of the lateral geniculate bodies. But various branches leave the tract before this point and go to other nuclei at the base of the brain. The branch which goes to the superior colliculi (CS) is important for spatial vision; from there branches pass to the centres for eye movements, but also to the peristriate areas, passing the striate area on the way (Fig. 4.16 below).

The *lateral geniculate body* (Fig. 4.13, *lateral geniculate nucleus*, LGN) is an accumulation of nerve cells the size of a peanut and consists of six layers, two 'magnocellular,' composed of large cells and four 'parvocellular' of small cells. As this organ lies beyond the chiasma, the left LGN represents the right half of the visual field and the right LGN the left half. The function of the LGN is still uncertain; neither the degree of binocular interaction nor the function of the magnocelluar and parvocellular systems has been fully elucidated. I shall return to that later.

The *optic radiation* (RO, Fig. 4.12, *radiatio optica*) contains the greatest number of optic fibres and is therefore indicated by a large arrow in Figure 4.16 below. The optic radiation is so called because the optic fibres fan out before they reach their following goal: the cerebral cortex of the occipital lobe of the brain.

The *striate area* is an area in which a white stripe, discovered by Gennari, can be seen with the naked eye. The visual cortex, about 3 mm thick, is divided into six layers (Fig. 4.14). The fibres of the optic radiation end in the fourth layer, on Gennari's line. The striate area is called the 'primary visual area' (area V1). It is the point of origin of fibres that run to other visual areas in the cerebral cortex.

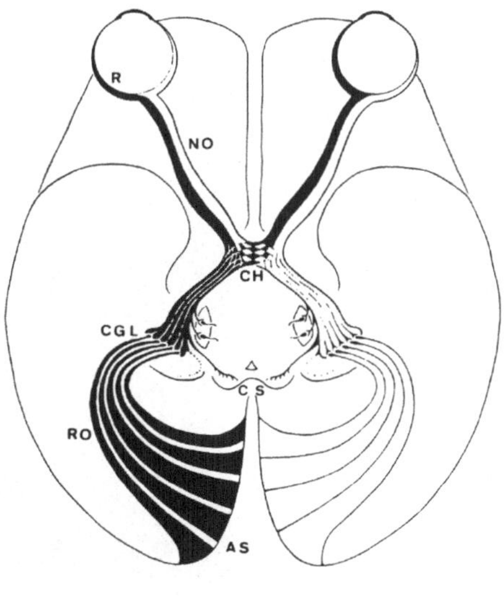

Fig. 4.12. From eye to area striata (Polyak, 1957). (R) Retina; (NO) optic nerve; (CH) chiasma; (CGL) lateral geniculate body; (RO) optic radiation; (AS) area striata; (CS) superior colliculi.

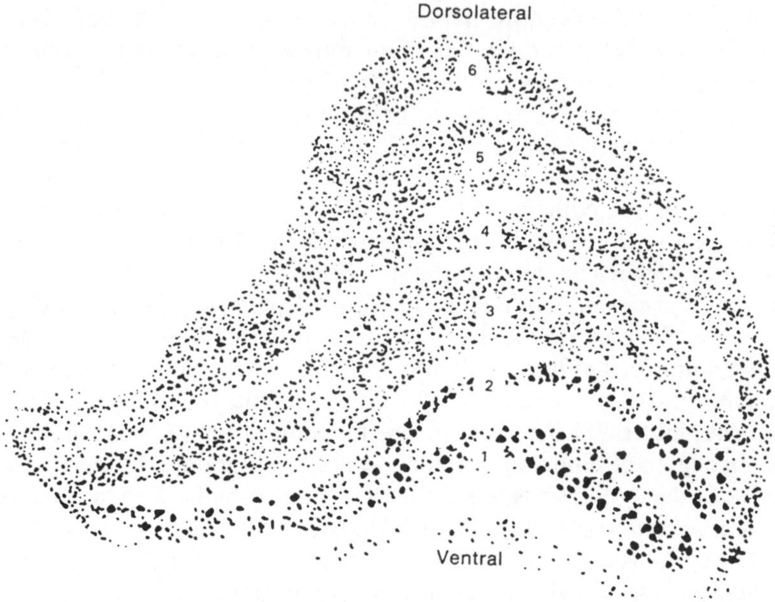

Fig. 4.13. Cross-section of lateral geniculate nucleus with its two magnocellular and four parvocellular layers. Each layer contains a map of the contralateral visual field (Carter, 1972).

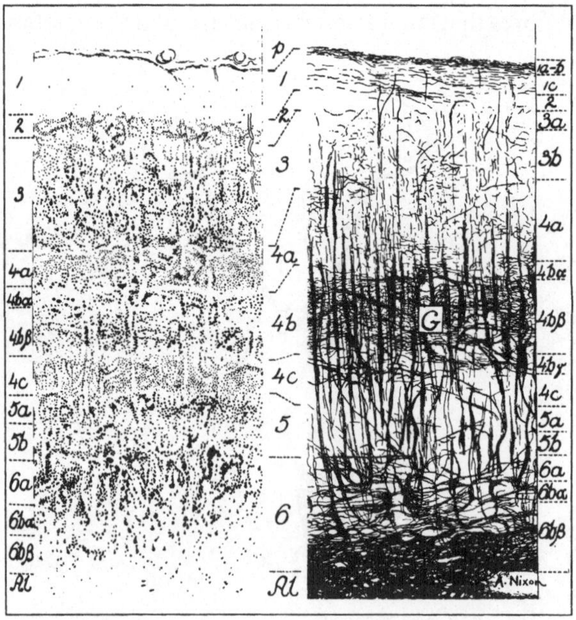

Fig. 4.14. Section of the visual cortex. On the left, the cell bodies of the neurons are stained, on the right the nerve fibres are made visible by a different method. (G) Gennari's line.

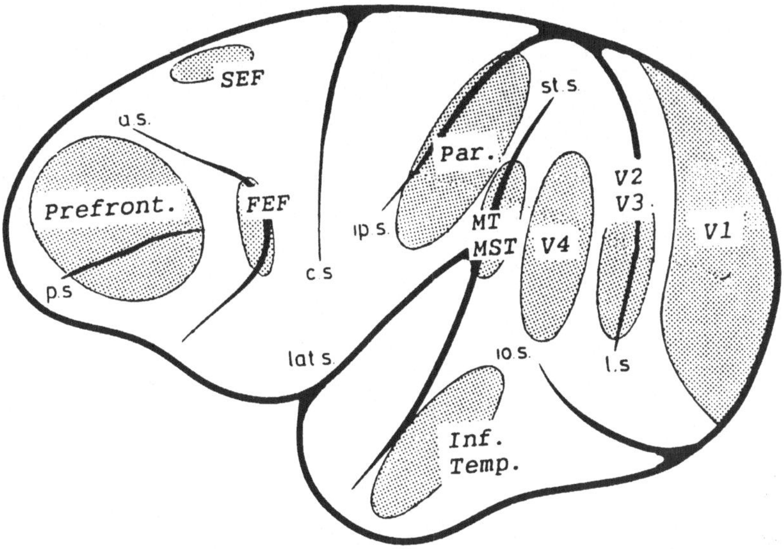

Fig. 4.15. Schematic drawing of the left hemisphere of a rhesus monkey's brain. (V1) Area striata; (V2,V3,V4) prestriatal visual areas; (MT) medial temporal cortex (V5); (MST) middle superior temporal cortex; (FEF) frontal eye field; (SEF) supplementary eye field. Shaded areas: prefrontal, parietal and inferotemporal cortex (Fischer & Boch, 1991).

The *prestriate area*, which is subdivided into areas V2,V3 and V4, receives the fibres from the striate area for further processing. Area V4 is responsible for colour vision. Physiological research in the rhesus monkey has revealed numerous secondary visual cortical areas (Fig. 4.15). Various visual cortical areas are also known in man. This knowledge has mainly been obtained by post-mortem examination of neurological patients. As can be seen in Fig. 4.16, the fibres fan out from the peristriate area in two main directions. Pathway II goes to the temporal cortex, pathway III to the parietal area.

The *temporal cortex* plays an important part in the recognition and naming of objects. Because of this, pathway II is called the 'what?'-pathway. The areas MT and MTS are specialised in the processing of information about movement.

The *parietal cortex* (especially areas 5 and 7) are important for spatial localization. Pathway III is therefore called the 'where?'-pathway. There must naturally be a close connection between the pathways II and III: if the parietal lobe localises something in a certain place, and the temporal lobe recognizes a horse, it is important to know that it is the horse which is in that particular place.

The *frontal cortex* is concerned with consciousness, emotions and personality. The frontal eye fields are the centres for voluntary movements. Afferent fibres mainly derive from the parietal and temporal cortex. Efferent fibres go to the superior colliculi, but also straight to the motor centres in the brain stem.

The *superior colliculi* have a key position in the control of eye movements. They are layered structures. The superficial layers receive fibres from numerous visual

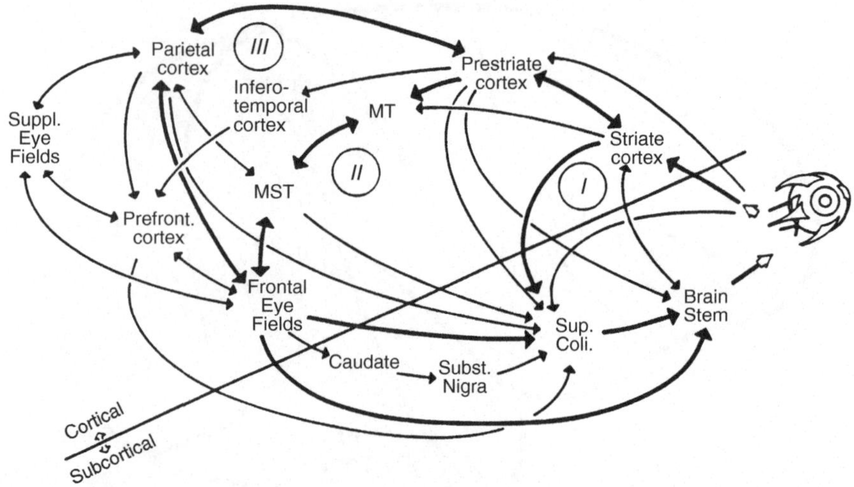

Fig. 4.16. The pathways involved in eye movements. The thick arrows emphasize three hypothetical loops (indicated by I, II and III), associated with different functional aspects of the preparation, generation and control of eye movements (Fischer & Boch, 1991).

areas. They are only small organs but it is thought that they process all the information of the 'where?' of visual objects, about their position in the visual field. In the deeper layers of the superior colliculi, auditory and somatosensory information is coupled with visual information. Some of the efferent motor fibres go to the oculomotor centres in the brain stem which innervate the eye muscles.

The *brain stem and cerebellum* control the visual eye movements and also coordinate the visual and vestibular impulses which lead to eye movements. We need not go into the details of these functions.

Figures 4.12 and 4.16 have been our guides in the preceding pages. The schematic representation in Figure 4.16 is, according to its compilers, 'too simple to account for a real monkey brain, yet too complex for *our* brain to understand even such simple things as eye movements.' We have adopted their material without question, but it is worth while explaining how all this knowledge has been acquired.

A SHORT HISTORY OF NEURAL LOCALISATION[2]

At first sight the brain is an amorphous, pulp-like mass. The ancient Egyptians already knew that and, while embalming mummies, sucked the brain out of the cranial cavity through the nose. The brain has managed to keep its secret for a long time. It is true that the Pythagorean Alkmaion (from Croton, 500 BC) considered the brain to be the 'seat' of our feelings, but great Aristotle thought that the function of the brain was to cool the blood. Galen, who lived a few hundred years later (but based his theories on Hippocrates and the early Alexandrian anatomists), and whose authority was unchallenged until the Renaissance, thought on the other

[2] Polyak, 1957; Brazier, 1984.

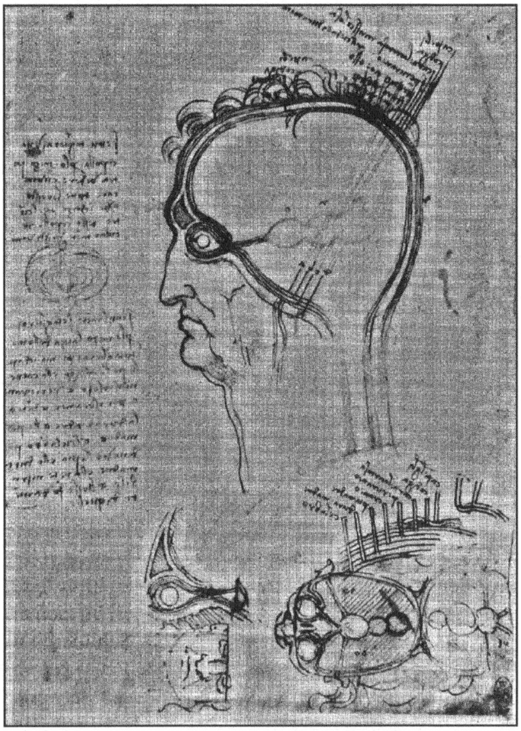

Fig. 4.17. The two optic nerves end in three successive brain cavities, which represent sensation, thought and memory. Drawing by Leonardo da Vinci (±1490) before he had discovered the real shape of the cavities by his own investigations (Strong, 1979).

hand that the brain was the *hegemonikon*, the controlling centre of the physical and spiritual individual. To cool the fiery heart, was the function of the respiration. Galen described the optic nerves as hollow. He thought that they communicated with each other in the chiasma, and in this way explained how the two eyes saw one image. He called the structure where the optic nerves enter the brain the *thalamus opticus*, the visual chamber.

In the Middle Ages the cavities of the brain received the most attention. That little can be stored in a cavity filled with liquid seems a disadvantage in our eyes, but for the Christian theorists it was more an advantage than otherwise: of course the soul could not be represented by a solid structure! Various aspects of the soul were localised in various brain cavities; thus sensory affections, logical thought and memory all had their own brain cavities. This mediaeval localisation theory, based on pure imagination, held its ground until the Renaissance (Fig. 4.17).

Descartes made a complete break with mediaeval theories and radically separated the material from the mental. He designed a plan of the visual pathways (Fig. 4.18), which was also pure conjecture. Theories about the visual pathways and their destination in the brain than stagnated for a long time. There were weighty philosophical objections to a visual centre in the brain. If the soul was an entity, the brain

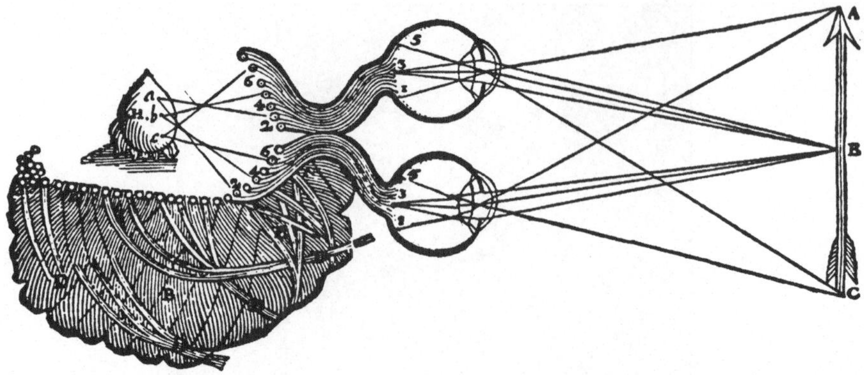

Fig. 4.18. Vision according to Descartes. Each retina projects onto the wall of the brain cavity. The projections are united in the pineal body (Descartes, 1664).

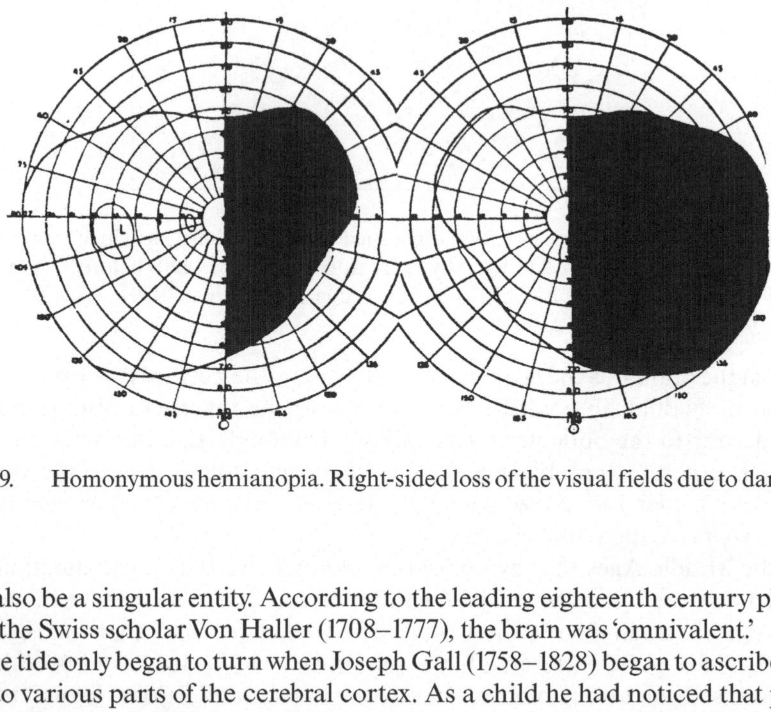

Fig. 4.19. Homonymous hemianopia. Right-sided loss of the visual fields due to damage to

must also be a singular entity. According to the leading eighteenth century physiologist, the Swiss scholar Von Haller (1708–1777), the brain was 'omnivalent.'

The tide only began to turn when Joseph Gall (1758–1828) began to ascribe functions to various parts of the cerebral cortex. As a child he had noticed that people with good memories had protruding eyes. He thought that exceptional development of certain talents could be discerned on the outside of the skull. In this way he was able to distinguish 27 different brain functions! Gall made the idea of specific functional localisations in the brain acceptable to the scientific world. His 'phrenology' maintained its popularity until well into the nineteenth century.

French neurologists and neuro-anatomists were the first to provide convincing arguments that the cerebral cortex was anything but omnivalent. An important step forward in our knowledge of the visual representation in the brain was made by the French neuro-anatomist Gratiolet. In 1857 he dissected the 'optic radiation' (which bears his name), leading from the LGN to the occipital cortex. Damage to the optic radiation is a common medical occurrence. Someone with a stroke, a large haemorrhage in one half of the brain, often has, in addition to paralysis of one side of the body, loss of half of the visual field (Fig. 4.19).

The discovery of the optic radiation made it clear that the occipital lobe plays an important part in vision. That was confirmed by physiological tests. Monkeys, whose occipital cortex had been removed, became blind. It is the striate area which is indispensable for vision.

Knowledge of the brain was obtained slowly and with difficulty until in the twentieth century an explosion of discovery took place. This was due to the refinement of neurological and neuropathological diagnosis and to animal experiments. The latter included anatomical tracing techniques (e.g., wth radio-active material) and histochemical methods, which made the nervous pathways microscopically visible; further, study of the motor effects of electrical stimulation of the brain, study of abormal behaviour following lesions, and finally—during visual stimulation—the tapping of neuronal action potentials by means of electrodes inserted into the brain substance. In all these ways we have learned a great deal, but we have also learned that we are still unable to understand the majority of the enormously complicated processes taking place in our brains.

5. The Evolution of the Eye and the Movements of the Eye[1]

THE EVOLUTION OF THE EYE

When we go back as far as possible in the phylogeny of the vertebrates, we arrive at the primitive Cyclostomata, eel-like creatures with eyes which, unfortunately from our point of view, demonstrate few fundamental differences from the eyes of less primitive vertebrates. The structure of the eyeball is like that of the human eye, and it is also moved by six muscles.

We can hardly go further back in the phylogeny. There is no creature living now from which we can deduce with certainty how the vertebrates evolved from more primitive organisms. Nevertheless, we can try to form a picture of the 'provertebrates' without skeletons, the ancestors of our fishes, by studying the individual development, the ontogeny, of the vertebrate embryo. The nineteenth-century biologist and philosopher Haeckel stated that the development of the egg-cell into the adult organism (the ontogeny) is a facsimile of the evolution (the phylogeny), by means of which the sort, in millions of years, has developed out of primitive life forms. His 'biogenetic law,' as formulated here, has proved to be incorrect, but to some degree it is possible to draw conclusions about ancestors from the embryonic forms of their descendants. For the study of eye movements and spatial vision, the evidence of ontogeny is not to be despised.

Figure 5.1 shows the ontogeny of the vertebrate eye. When the human embryo is less than 3 mm long the neural plate appears on its back. The front part, from which the brain will later develop, is largely occupied by the first rudiments of the retinas. The eye thus develops on the upper surface of the embryo. The neural plate later becomes the neural tube, while the brain develops between the rudimentary retinas. The primitive retina, which now forms the optic vesicle, has not yet lost contact with the skin. In the five-week, 11 mm embryo it invaginates and forms an optic cup, while the skin above it forms a lens. The brain gradually comes to occupy a deeper, safer position, while remaining attached to the eyes by the optic nerves, which are at first hollow.

[1] Walls, 1942; Polyak, 1957; Duke-Elder, 1958; Crone, 1973; Sarnat and Netsky, 1974; Cronly-Dillon and Gregory, 1991.

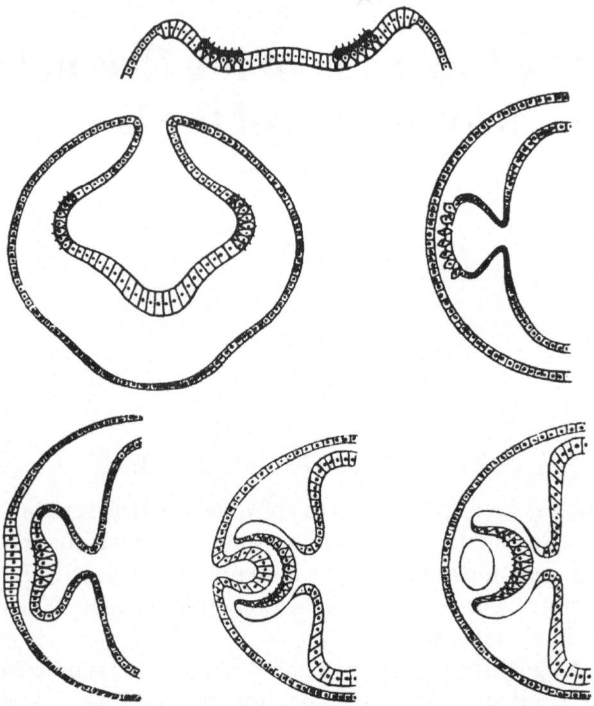

Fig. 5.1. The ontogenesis of the vertebrate eye (Duke-Elder, 1958).

We may imagine that the eye of our distant invertebrate ancestor has evolved along the same lines as the embryo's eye. Guesses like this are justified because we see the same primitive developmental stages in other, still living, creatures. An example is the snail, some types of which have only a bundle of light-sensitive cells in the skin, while others have real eyes with lenses, like those found in vertebrate eyes (Fig. 5.2).

The provertebrate will have been a limp water creature, that may have lived at the bottom of shallow pools. That would explain why the organs with which stimuli were received and processed, the so-called sensory organs, were situated on its back. Light-sensitive cells developed there, on the right and left sides. For such primitive defenceless creatures, light stimuli (passing shadows and flashes of light produced by light-reflecting animals) will not have signified much more than approaching danger. Stimulation of the light-sensitive organs will only have produced an escape reaction. Escape meant: turn your head the other way and swim in a different direction; in other words, contract the side of the body opposite to the stimulated eye (Fig. 5.3). Thus, a special relationship developed between the eye as 'nociceptor' (detector of harmful things) and the contralateral side of the body, a relationship which we see manifested in the crossing of the optic nerves, the chiasma, which is encountered in all vertebrates.

Only later, when the eye had developed so far that it could form real images, did the optic stimuli have more significance for the animal than merely the signal to

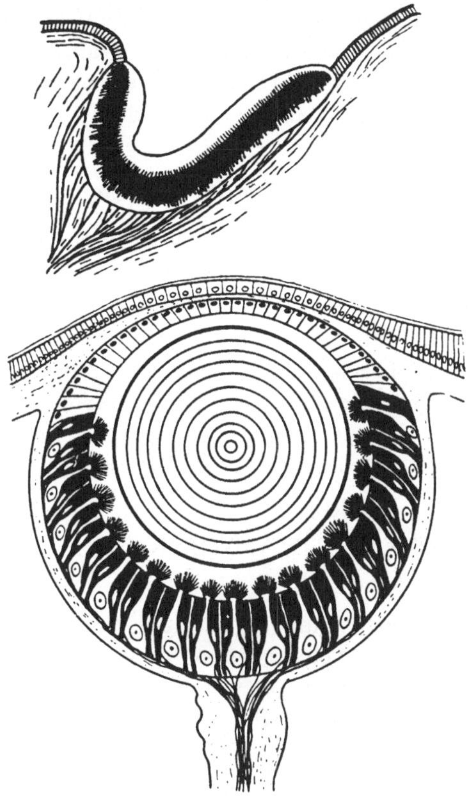

Fig. 5.2. Stages in the phylogenetic development of the snail eye. Above: *Patella*; below: *Helix* (Polyak, 1957).

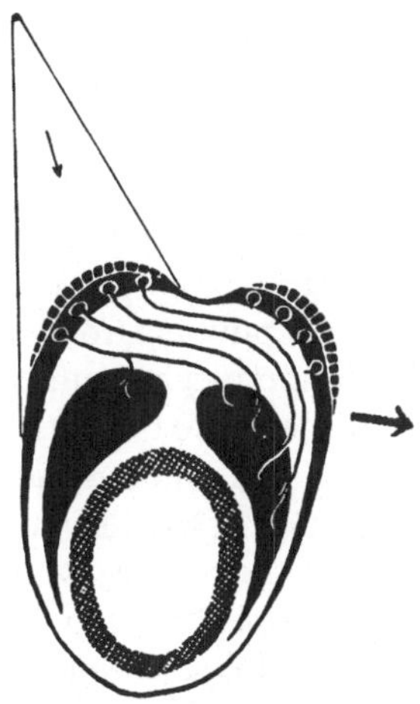

Fig. 5.3. Negative optotaxis. Hypothetical relation between sensory epithelium and contralateral musculature (Polyak, 1957).

escape. Only then was it possible to distinguish between a danger signal and unthreatening visual stimuli, which finally would obtain the significance of 'prey.' The more highly developed eye could thus acquire a new biological function and become part of the attacking mechanism.

THE EVOLUTION OF THE EYE MOVEMENTS

We had to go back to the snail for an idea of how the vertebrate eye, that has almost completed its development in the most primitive fish, could have developed. An important premise is that the eye movements needed by an eye with a mainly nociceptive (danger signalling) function differ from those needed by a 'positively optotactic,' prey-detecting eye. The optic danger-detector must be able to distinguish a moving hostile object from the stationary environment, so that the animal can escape. The prey-detector has a double task: to recognize prey, which is often moving, and to keep it fixated while leading the animal's body to the prey.

COMPENSATORY MOVEMENTS AND BINOCULAR OPTOMOTOR REFLEXES

To detect danger, the eye must be able to distinguish between moving and stationary objects. This is a comparatively easy task for an animal which does not move itself, a task which does not involve the eye muscles. The situation is different for a moving, wriggling creature. If the eyes did not move in a moving head, the image of the outside world would flash continually back and forth over the retina and it would be impossible to distinguish a moving source of danger from the moving environment. That is only possible if the eyes are maintained in a constant position in relation to the outside world. Paradoxically enough, the first eye movements served to keep the eyes stationary in relation to the outside world. These movements, which the most primitive fishes are capable of, were initiated by the labyrinths and the proprioceptive organs in the neck. Because movements in three directions more or less at right angles to each other were necessary for adequate compensation (Fig. 5.4), all vertebrates had from the start three pairs of eye muscles on each eye. Although supplemented by other types of movement, compensatory movements have remained of paramount importance, even in man.

At an early stage in the phylogeny, *optic* environment-fixating reflexes were added to the vestibular and proprioceptive environment-fixating reflexes, resulting in improvement in the immobilisation mechanism of the eye. The afferent part of these reflexes ran through the optic nerves to the optic lobes in the brain stem, which in turn became connected with the oculomotor pathways between the labyrinths and the eye muscles. Every stimulation of the vestibular organ by turning the head was accompanied by stimulation of the retinas, where the images of the environment moved over them both in the same direction. The visual and non-visual oculomotor reflexes became automatically adjusted to each other. Thus optic and labyrinthine reflexes both contributed to the stabilisation of the image; they made use of a common pathway to the motor nuclei for the eye muscles, which are responsible for identical *conjugated* movements of the eyes.

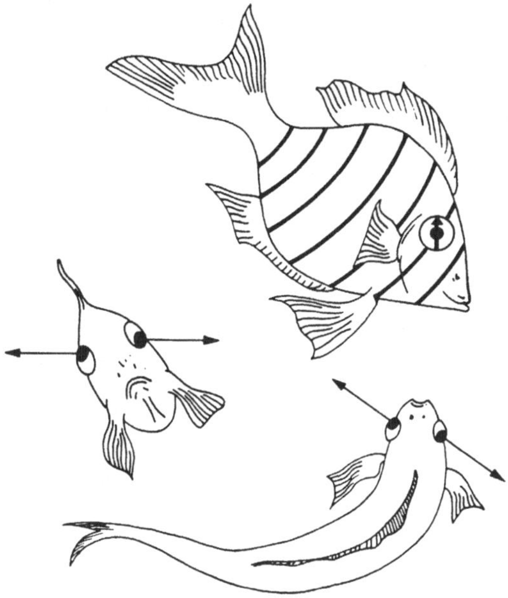

Fig. 5.4. Compensatory eye movements.

Of course there are limits to the mobility of the eyes. When a fish makes a wide turn to the left its eyes make a compensatory turn to the right until the limit of the eyes' mobility is reached. The eyes then make a rapid jerk back to the middle position and the slow, environment-fixating, turn to the right begins again. This continual alternation of slow movements and rapid recovery movements in the opposite direction is called 'nystagmus.' It was originally a vestibular mechanism but, because of the secondary connection between vestibular and visual stimuli described above, nystagmus has an optical component also.

The connection between the vestibular and the visual stimuli can be broken experimentally. Isolated stimulation of the labyrinth can be obtained, for instance, by caloric stimulation (cold water in the external ear); pure 'vestibular nystagmus' is then produced. On the other hand, the head can be kept still, so that the labyrinths are not stimulated, and a figure, such as a pattern of vertical stripes, can be moved about in front of the eyes. That produces 'optokinetic nystagmus.' Both forms of nystagmus consist of a slow environment-fixating phase and a quick jerky recovery movement, the so-called 'saccade.' In higher vertebrates we see these two phases as the slow following movement and the rapid gaze movement. In this way the vestibular-optokinetic system is the basis of all sorts of conjugate eye movements.

MONOCULAR EYE MOVEMENTS

So far, the vestibular and optical environment-fixating reflexes have been considered which are necessary for the eye as a danger-detecting organ. The optical prey detector, however, has different requirements. The animal must be led to its prey.

For this purpose it is necessary—especially in the case of swift pursuers—that the moving prey is fixated and not the stationary environment. As soon as a potential victim is sighted, the vestibular and optic compensatory reflexes must give way to the optic prey-fixating reflexes. There is one fundamental difference between the compensatory reflexes needed for the fixation of the environment and the eye movements necessary for the fixation of the prey: when an animal moves its head, the image of its surroundings moves simultaneously over the two retinas; thus vestibular compensatory movements are always *binocular.* But when an animal sights its prey, its image will usually only fall on one retina, because the eyes of most primitive vertebrates are implanted laterally and have little communal visual field. The fixation of the prey will therefore initially be *monocular.* Only after the chase has started will the animal take up a position in which the prey is straight in front of both eyes.

In this way, two sorts of eye movements form the foundation of our optic motility: binocular reflexes, vestibular and optokinetic, on the one hand, and monocular fixation reflexes on the other hand, with their own motor pathway to the nuclei of the ocular muscles of one eye.

A number of factors determine which of these reflexes has the upper hand in a given animal species. In the case of plant-eating fish, which are mainly dependent on their sense of smell for finding food, the eye functions chiefly as part of an alarm system. For this purpose, stabilisation of the environment by vestibulo-ocular reflexes, together with a lateral position of the eyes which produces a panoramic visual field, is extremely important. The same considerations also apply to some more advanced animals, such as the rabbit. The situation is different when the eyes are indispensable for hunting prey. Monocular eye movements are then seen, at least in non-mammals. These can be clearly observed in predatory fish, especially fish like seahorses, pike and the inhabitants of coral reefs, that normally remain motionless, a condition which makes fewer demands on binocular stabilisation (although vestibulo-ocular reflexes also remain indispensable in those animals).

THE FOVEA AND THE VISUAL FIXATION OF PREY

A characteristic feature of all animals that make spontaneous fixation movements is the presence of a fovea, a highly differentiated retinal area on which the object which forms the stimulus to fixation is projected by means of a fixation movement. The more highly developed the spontaneous eye movements are, as expression of a way of life concentrated on small or distant prey, the better the fovea is differentiated. An excellent example is the highly developed fovea of the chameleon. This reptile sits immobile on a branch watching for small insects. As its body does not move, binocular, conjugated eye movements are not necessary. The eyes make completely independent searching movements (Fig. 5.5). Whenever an object that is projected on the periphery of the retina attracts attention, an eye movement takes place which causes the image to fall on the fovea. This movement is extremely precise and its direction and amplitude is determined by the position of the point of stimulation in the peripheral retina, because each retinal point has its own *local sign.*

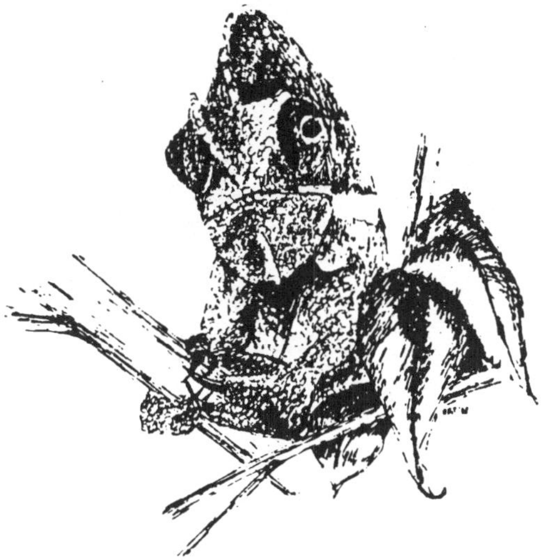

Fig. 5.5. Chameleon. Monocular searching movements.

BINOCULAR VISION AND CONVERGENCE IN THE CHAMELEON AND IN FISH

When the chameleon sees an insect, he directs his head and both eyes towards the prey and catches it by putting out his sticky, sucking tongue (Fig. 5.6). Here we encounter a new type of vision, binocular vision, and a new type of eye movement, convergence of the two eyes (assisted by efficient accommodation) onto the prey, which is localised straight in front of the head. *We must regard this convergence as a monocular movement carried out by both eyes at the same time.* The monocular movements in the two eyes are dissimilar because the starting positions of the two individually moving eyes are different.

When the eyes are both directed towards the prey, the visual axes of the eyes converge more strongly when the prey is close by and less strongly when the prey is further away. On the basis of the convergence (and the associated accommodation) the chameleon is able to estimate the distance in order to protrude his tongue to the right length. This requires intensive coordination of the optomotor impulses, originating from the two eyes, in the central nervous system. The most important central representation of the retinas is formed by the two optic lobes of the tectum opticum, structures projecting dorsally from the brain stem. These paired structures have fibre connections with each other and with the telencephalon, the forerunner of our cerebral cortex.

Binocular vision also takes place in the median plane in some fish, despite their laterally placed eyes. When the prey approaches they direct their heads towards it. In both eyes the retinal images shift in the temporal direction. This induces a bilateral adduction of the eyes in order to focus the image on the foveae (Fig. 5.7). Binocular vision and binocular convergence are apparently so important for the animal that

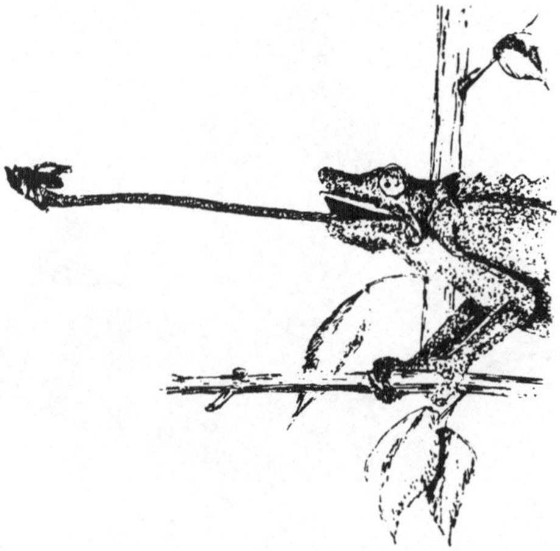

Fig. 5.6. Chameleon. Binocular convergence when prey is caught.

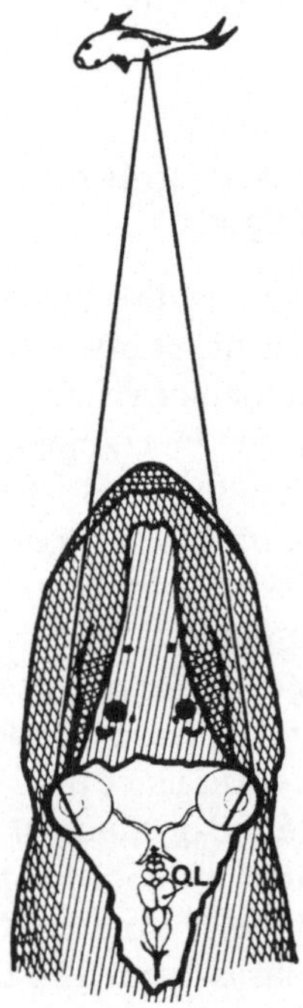

Fig. 5.7. Convergence of the eyes of a pike. The two eyes have been drawn schematically with the optic nerves, and the brain with the optic lobes (OL) (Polyak, 1957).

the definition of the image is sacrificed for it, at least in fish with laterally placed eyes. The 'foveae,' or at least the retinal areas with increased cell density which mediate binocular vision, are placed very eccentrically (Fig. 5.8), but their central representations meet in the optic lobes. The binocular estimation of distance achieved in

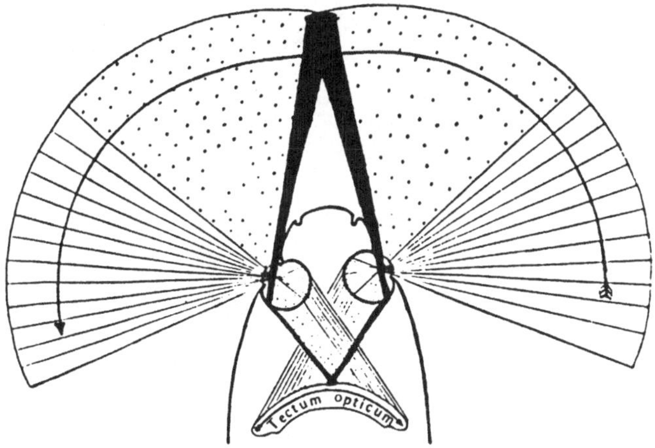

Fig. 5.8. Total decussation of the optic nerves in a fish with little more than panoramic vision. Note the convergence in the optic tectum of those fibres carrying impulses from the small portions of the visual fields that overlap (Kappers et al., 1936, after Sarnat & Netsky, 1974).

this way is undoubtedly far from perfect; it misses optic definition and is only effective in the median plane during convergence.

DEPTH VISION AND DISPARITY

In the evolution of vision and eye movements the further development of the distance response is of prime importance. Up till now the *convergence* was considered to be the oculomotor correlative of the distance response. In birds and mammals, however, there is a second, no less important, correlative, the so-called *disparity.* This concept will be discussed extensively in the chapter on depth vision; for the present moment it is enough to state that each eye sees a near object from its own viewpoint. Therefore, the two retinal images of a near object are slightly different, slightly 'disparate,' the more different the object comes nearer.

For the perception of small differences between the two retinal images the visual system has to meet two requirements:

1. *Frontally positioned eyes*: When the binocular field of vision is large, depth vision from disparity will be more successfull. Moreover, the optical quality of frontally placed eyes, when the fovea approaches the optical axis, is better, enabling the eyes to detect smaller inter-ocular differences.
2. *A close network of nerve fibres between the central projections of the two retinas*, making precise comparison possible between the signals from the two eyes, is the second requirment.

BINOCULAR VISION IN BIRDS

In the course of the evolution of their visual system, birds have found their own way to improve binocular vision. As an example, take the owl with its pronounced

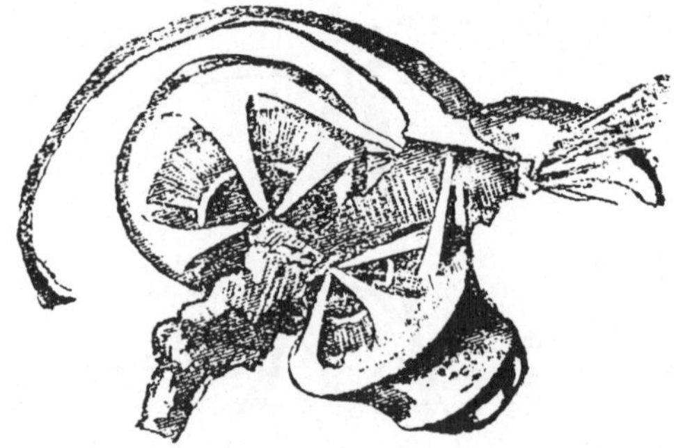

Fig. 5.9. Owl, dissected. Immobile eyes, underdeveloped oculomotor muscles (Motais, 1887).

frontal eyes. A remarkable, indeed unique feature of the owl is, that the eyes are quite immobile—and this despite the presence of (very underdeveloped) eye muscles (Fig. 5.9). Against this, however, the head is exceptionally mobile. Owls are nocturnal creatures and, like all in this category, have relatively poor visual acuity with a poorly developed area centralis. Because of this—and despite the immobility of the eyes—the bitemporal shift of the retinal image which occurs when an owl approaches its prey or another object, does not result in serious diminution of visual acuity.

Owls are incapable of convergence, yet this fact does not preclude depth perception. Anyone who has seen an owl flying at high speed between the trees in a dense forest can have no doubt as to its ability to perceive depth. That capacity is due to the partial double crossing of the tecto-telencephalic tract. Figure 5.10 shows that there is a complete crossing (decussation) of the optic nerves and a partial crossing (semidecussation) of the tecto-telencephalic tract. This leads to intensive contact between the corresponding projections of the two retinas, so that slight differences between the two retinal images can be detected and the binocular perception of depth becomes possible.

As early as 1917 Ariëns Kappers, the comparative neuro-anatomist, described the basic principle of neuro-anatomy, *neurobiotaxis*: neurons involved in an intense functional relationship move, in the course of evolution, towards each other so that their connections become as short as possible. This evolutionary process in some birds has resulted in the central representations of the retinas *coinciding after one total crossing of the optic nerves and a half crossing of the tecto-telencephalic tract.* Mammals have achieved this even more efficiently: by means of *partial crossing of the optic nerves themselves.*

DEPTH PERCEPTION AND THE SEMIDECUSSATION OF THE OPTIC NERVES IN MAMMALS: CORRESPONDING BINOCULAR POINTS

In mammals the evolution of the visual system is different. Most of the fibres of the optic nerves no longer go to the optic tectum, but to another important area in the

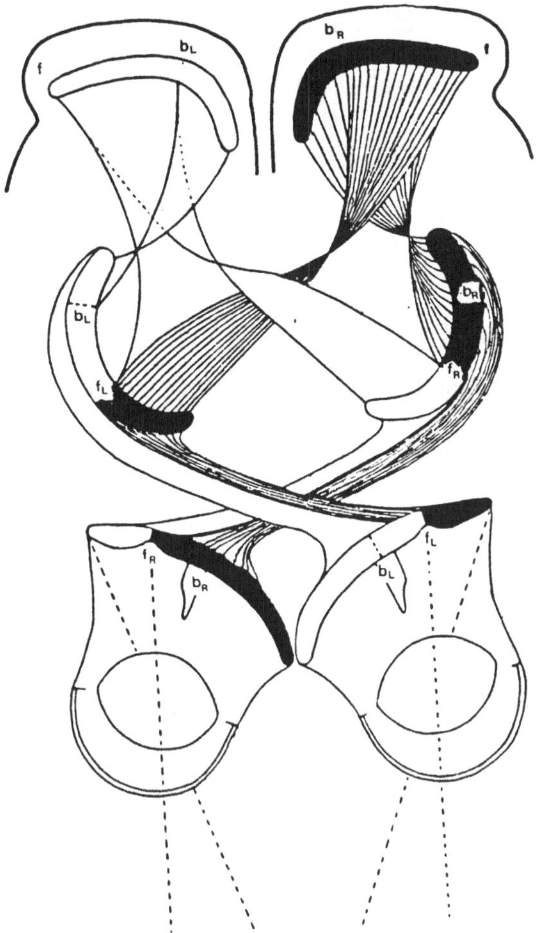

Fig. 5.10. Double decussation pattern which mediates binocular interaction in owls and some other predatory birds by means of a second decussation; information from corresponding parts of each retina converge in the brain. (f) The binocular fovea on the temporal retina and its representation in the central visual pathway. After Pettigrew (1991).

brain stem: the lateral geniculate nucleus. In addition, a *partial crossing* (*semidecussation*) *of the optic nerves takes place in the chiasma* (Fig. 4.12). The result of this partial crossing is that the central projections from the nasal half of the retina of one eye and the temporal half of the retina of the other eye (which together process the stimuli from one half of the visual field) lie close to each other in the cerebrum. This is already the case in the lateral geniculate nuclei, the first nuclei reached by the optic fibres in the brain stem. But these organs probably only play a minor part in binocular vision; they have an extensive projection to the cerebral cortex (Fig. 4.12). That is the place where stimuli deriving from one point in space, via the two eyes, meet in the brain: they are *corresponding points* (we concentrate at present on stimuli deriving from a distant point in space, in order to minimize the influence of the distance between the eyes). Traditionally one speaks of 'corresponding retinal points,' but it is really cortical elements which correspond with each other. It is better to speak of 'corresponding binocular points' than 'corresponding retinal points.'

The migration of the visual centre to the large visual area in the neocortex created an enormous amount of space in which binocular vision could develop further. Functions which in lower animals were performed by the retina, have been transferred to the cortex in mammals. The retina of a frog is able to track the path of a flying insect, a task that, in mammals, has been taken over by the visual cortex. 'Encephalisation' has taken place.

SEMIDECUSSATION AND CONJUGATE EYE MOVEMENTS

Through the semidecussation in the chiasma the coupling of the eyes has become so intense that binocular vision is continually in use. This has led to a fundamental change in the eye movements in mammals. While binocular vision in the pike, during the depth response, only corresponded with the movement of images *in opposite directions*, especially in the median plane, with convergence and divergence as the motor consequences, binocular movements in mammals are now also made *in the same direction*, when a fixated object is moving or attention is diverted to another object in the frontal plane. The efferent mechanism for these movements was already present in the mechanism of compensatory eye movements, that served to compensate parallel shifts of the image due to conjugated eye movements. It is therefore not surprising that optically conjugated eye movements, arising from corresponding binocular points, also make use of the nerve tracts preformed by the compensatory mechanism. Because of this, monocular motility, which had its own connections with the nuclei of the eye muscles, has been relegated to the background. Only convergence (and divergence, the relaxation of convergence) may be regarded as relics of monocular movements (and—perhaps—small disjunctive corrective movements in the vertical and torsional directions, although these may also have developed from compensatory vestibular eye movements).

While convergence was still asymmetrical in the chameleon because of the different initial positions of the eyes, in mammals it has become symmetrical through binocular coupling. This is called Hering's law. There are exceptions to this law, when convergence fails to succeed in hiding its monocular origin.

It is clear that the semidecussation is an important acquisition from the point of view of spatial vision. The close proximity of the projections of the two retinas allows small disparities (simultaneous stimulation of non-corresponding retinal points; for instance, bitemporal points stimulated by a near-by object) to be detected with great precision. However, the binocular vision available to man also has its disadvantages. The independently functioning eyes of the chameleon could carry out a visual search in the same way as two hands can search independently for something tangible. Our eyes, on the other hand, are coupled together. If anything interferes with that, we risk double vision.

6. Directional Vision

INTRODUCTION

The most important task of the eyes when exploring space is the identification of directions. The 'extensiveness,' which was considered by Descartes to be the essence of space, is provided with two of its three spatial dimensions by the perception of directions. The appropriate system for the description of these two directions is the polar co-ordinate system with its centre approximately at the turning-point of the head (the visual egocentre). The primary direction is straight ahead when the eyes are in the central position. One co-ordinate is the *direction* in relation to the primary direction (above-to the right-below-to the left), the other is the *eccentricity* in relation to the primary direction. These co-ordinates determine the surveyable visual space. The visual perception of space is the start of a sensorimotor process which ends with the strike of a claw or the snap of teeth. In primitive animals the surveyable part of space is identical with the 'field of visually-directed motor action.' As the animal's visuomotor system becomes better developed, more intermediate links appear between perception and action. Action can be delayed, altered or cancelled.

In man, the orientation towards a visual object has a *psychological* correlate in the 'egocentric localisation.' That is the localisation of a visual object in subjective space in relation to the visual egocentre. The subjective vertical median plane runs through this point, and is—together with the horizontal plane—an important point of reference in psychological space. The subjective optic median plane coincides with the objective median plane when the eyes are directed forwards in the position of physiological rest. Although it is impossible in animals to speak of a directional localisation without motor action, in humans this is possible. For example, a chess player can localise a piece adequately on C6 without pointing to it.

DIRECTIONAL VISION AND EYE MOVEMENTS[1]

In the previous chapter I have tried to demonstrate that the complicated organisation of binocular vision has developed from simpler forms existing in non-mammals. These simpler types of organisation form the starting point for the following observations. The situation in animals is considered under A and in humans under B.

[1] Crone, 1973.

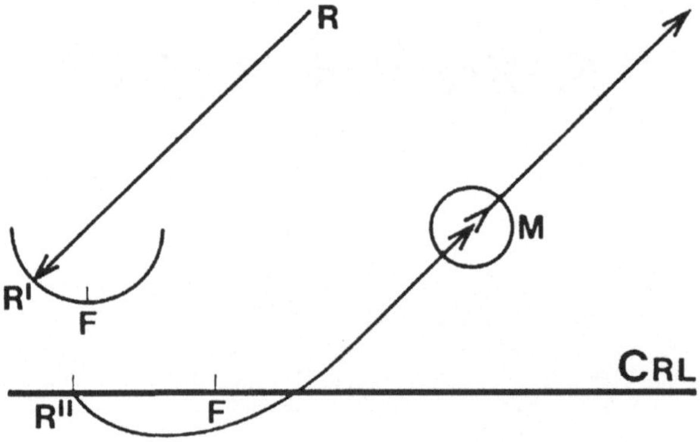

Fig. 6.1. Directional orientation and retinal local sign. (F) Fovea; (R) visual object on the right; (R′) retinal image of this object; (R″) central representation of this object; (M) motor centre for movements of the animal; (CRL) central representation of the retinas.

RETINAL LOCAL SIGNS

(A) For an animal which is lying still and not moving its eyes, visual directional localisation is a simple task. The position of the object is then determined by the position of the retinal image, the 'local sign,' only. When such an animal sees its prey to the right, it only has to stretch its leg out to the right, an action that is regulated by a motor stimulus arising from point R″ of the central representation of the retina, from which a motor impulse is sent to the claw (Fig. 6.1). The relation between the retina and the claw only appears to be immediate: the neural pathway from the retina to the claw traverses the central representation of the retina and—presumably—the neural centre for conjugate eye movements.

(B) A similar situation to that described above can occur in humans. If someone who is reading a book in the garden sees an insect in his right visual field, he can wave it away with his hand without interrupting his reading.

THE INFLUENCE OF COMPENSATORY EYE MOVEMENTS ON DIRECTIONAL VISION

(A) Fish, rabbits and other animals have no, or hardly any, spontaneous eye movements, but move their eyes under the influence of stimuli arising in the labyrinths and the muscles of the neck. In such animals adequate motor reactions are not determined by the position of the retinal image only. This is illustrated in Figure 6.2. When the head is turned to the left, and the eyes (by a compensatory reflex) to the right, space does not move in relation to the retina, but it does move in relation to the snout. The foveae are now stimulated by an object that does not lie straight in front of the snout but to the right of it. *For an adequate reaction a change is needed in the relation between the local sign and the action, which is quantitatively the same as the compensatory change in the position of the eyes.*

(B) It is not easy in humans to study quantitatively the compensatory change in localisation that takes place under the influence of postural factors. The motility of

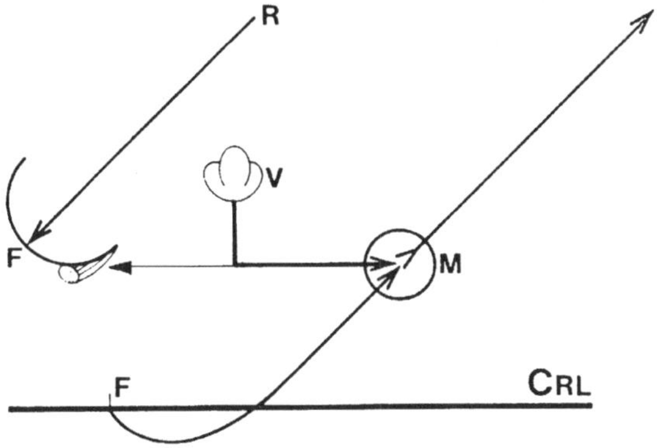

Fig. 6.2. Directional localization and compensatory deviation of the eyes. Same abbreviations as in Figure 6.1. (V) Vestibular and proprioceptive apparatus, which moves the eyes to the right when the head turns to the left. Now object R, that is imaged on the fovea, is not localized straight ahead, but to the right.

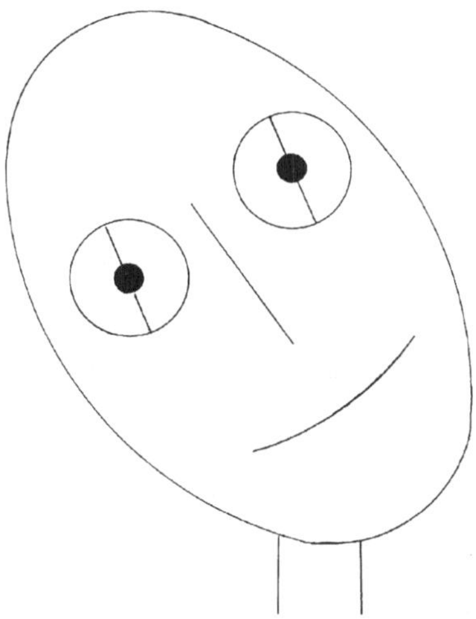

Fig. 6.3. Compensatory countertorsion of the eyes when the head is tilted.

the human eye is so largely determined by voluntary gaze movements that it is difficult to determine the resting position and the deviations from that position due to vestibular reflexes. Only cycloversions, the torsional movements of the eyes round their optic axes, are completely reflectory. When the head turns round the sagittal axis there is a compensatory rolling of the eyes in the opposite direction (Fig. 6.3). The change in position of the subjective median plane is quantitatively the same as the compensatory rolling of the eyes (Fig. 6.4). In other words, space remains stable in relation to the eyes, but not in relation to the head.

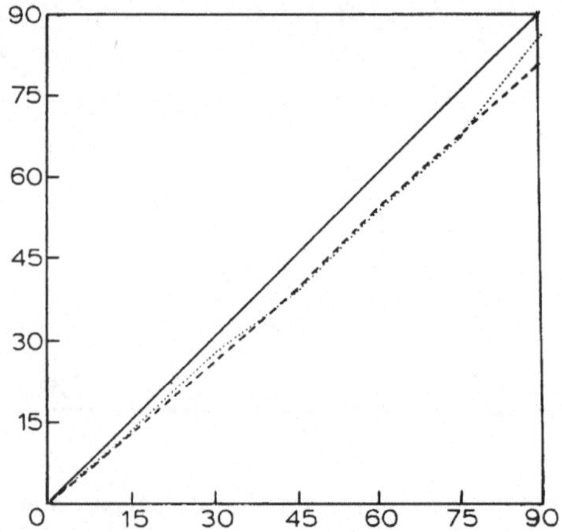

Fig. 6.4. Quantitative equivalence of compensatory countertorsion and rotation of the subjective medial plane. Horizontal axis: rotation of the head around a sagittal axis (degrees). Vertical axis: rotation (degrees) of vertical retinal meridian (. . .) and subjective medial plane (– – –) (Mesker, 1953).

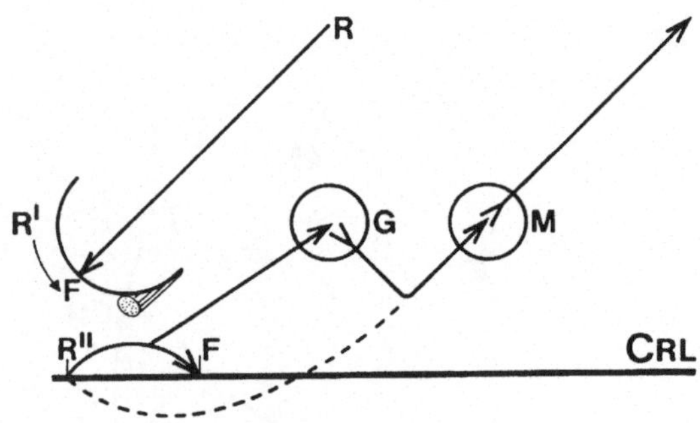

Fig. 6.5. Directional orientation and saccadic movements. Same abbreviations as in Figure 6.1. R initially stimulates R′. Broken line: localization according to local sign. After the saccade the localization has been taken over by G, the centre for movements of gaze.

INFLUENCE OF GAZE MOVEMENTS

(A) In animals with spontaneous gaze movements, visual localisation becomes still more complicated. In Figure 6.5, object R originally falls on a non-foveal retinal point R′. It is possible that the animal may not fixate point R. Certainly no rapidly moving animal will direct its gaze towards every passing obstacle. We then have a similar situation to that of animals with only compensatory eye movements. But it is also possible that the eye (the fovea) will be directed towards point R. *The retinal signal 'right front' is then ended, but replaced by an apparently equivalent signal 'gaze directed towards right front.'* Again the correct orientation is obtained with the help of an intermediate station between the retinal local sign and the centre for body motility, namely, a centre for voluntary gaze movements.

This confronts us with an important fact in the theory of directional vision: the *equivalence of the retinal local sign and the gaze movement*: it doesn't matter whether the directional localisation occurs via a peripheral retinal point or through a gaze innervation, a foveating eye movement. In Figure 6.5 point R remains in front and to the right before and after the gaze movements. During gaze movements the field of visual action does not shift. The centre of that field remains straight ahead and the field is scanned by gaze movements.

(B) The same applies to humans. When the position of the eyes changes because of a voluntary gaze movement, subjectively everything stays in the same place. When we move our gaze from straight ahead to 20 degrees to the right, two things happen. In the first place, the image of the complete visual world shifts to the left over the retina. Nevertheless, we see no movement: the shift takes place too quickly for movement to be seen and, in addition, vision is to some extent suppressed during the saccade. But the second fact is still more extraordinary: after the saccade the visual world has not shifted! The local sign of the peripheral point (20 degrees to the right) is apparently annexed by the fovea centralis.

If we apply pressure to our eyes we see space shift. If we stimulate the labyrinths by spouting cold water into the outer ear, the world turns. Passive and reflex movements do produce displacement of our visual world, but active, voluntary gaze movements leave the perceptual space in position. There have been many speculations, mostly fruitless, about how this can be. It has been thought that space must 'really' shift during gaze movements, and mechanisms have been devised by which this would be prevented. For an adequate explanation the physiological difference between active and reflex movements would have to be defined and, in addition, not only visual space but also multimodal perceptual space would have to be included. At present we can only conclude that *reflex and voluntary eye movements have different influences on our directional vision.*

DIRECTIONAL VISION WITH TWO EYES

As long as the eyes are directed towards distance and are stimulated by an object in the distance the directional localisation with two eyes is the same as when only one eye is being used. But when a near object is fixated in the median plane, the right eye is directed towards the left and the left eye to the right. The directional localisation of the object is not determined by the position of one or the other eye, but is straight in front. If the image of a near object at one side falls on the eyes, the situation is represented by Figure 6.6. The directional localisation is again intermediate and the direction of R is not determined by R's local sign in either the right or the left eye. *During convergence the directional localisation is intermediate.* The full explanation of this fact will be given in Chapter 7.

THE RANGE OF DIRECTIONAL VISION

The range of directional vision is determined by three factors: the size of the visual field (in immobile eyes), the mobility of the eyes themselves and the mobility of the neck.

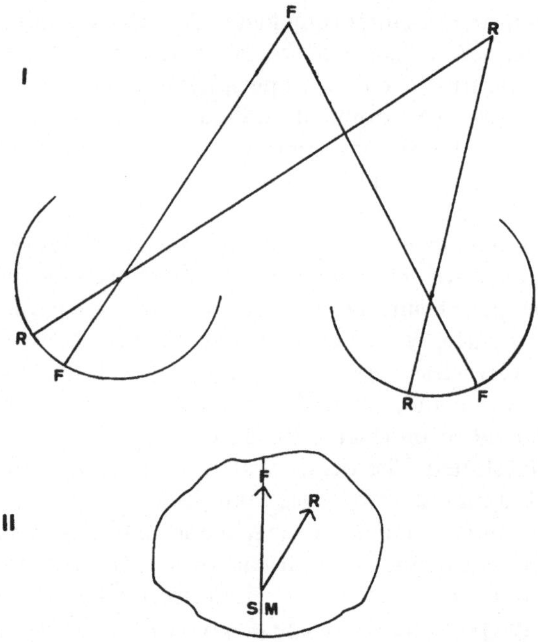

Fig. 6.6. Binocular vision and the intermediate localisation of direction. (I) the retinal distance R–F is greater in the right eye than in the left eye. (II) R is seen in space in the intermediate direction. (SM) subjective medial plane.

The mobility of human eyes is great, as much as 50 degrees in the sideways direction. When the attention is attracted by a peripheral object, the eye makes a rapid saccade which may be accompanied by a rapid head movement. Subsequently the movement of the eyes usually decreases and the turning of the head becomes correspondingly greater. The first phase of the head-and-eye movement is often called a *gaze movement*; the second phase resembles a vestibulo-ocular reflex, but is more or less voluntary. A girl who wants to let her boy friend, and him alone, see that she is looking at him, keeps her head still and looks archly out of the corner of her eye; on the other hand, someone who doesn't want to give the impression that he is prying, looks straight ahead and only moves his head. In many animals the range of eye movements is smaller than in man. When a cat looks at you it is its head that is directed towards you. The owl, whose cylindrical eyes cannot turn, performs gaze movements by turning its head only.

THE VISUAL FIELD

In animals with laterally placed eyes, like the rabbit, the visual field of both eyes is panoramic. Such a large visual field guarantees safety when flight is the only weapon, but is almost entirely monocular, so that stereoscopic vision is hardly done justice to. Beasts of prey have a smaller visual field, but an important part of it is binocular (Fig. 6.7). In humans too the greater part of the visual field is binocular.

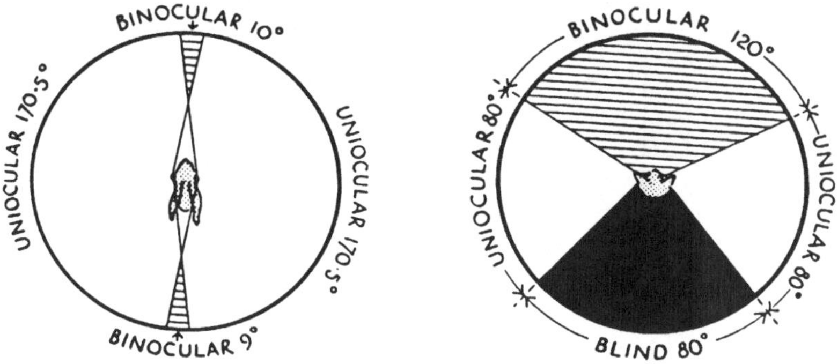

Fig. 6.7. Visual fields of rabbit and cat (Duke-Elder, 1958).

The measurement of the visual field is important in ophthalmology. Therefore there are sensitive instruments for the detection of even the smallest defect. In *projection perimeters* a spot of light of carefully controlled brightness is projected onto the inside of a hemisphere, while the patient looks at a fixation light at the centre. A large, bright spot of light is used for the 'absolute boundary' of the visual field. As the sensitivity to small spots of light gradually increases from the periphery to the fovea, the use of increasingly weak lights produces increasingly narrow 'relative' boundaries to the visual field. These relative boundaries are an artefact of the examination method, but have a successful existence in ophthalmological diagnostics. Careless examinations can lead to curious mistakes (Fig. 6.8).

THE CHARTING OF THE VISUAL FIELD IN THE BRAIN

In Chapter 4 some basic facts about neuro-anatomy and neurophysiology were given, in so far as they were related to the visual system. The starting-point was the fundamental diagram shown in Figure 4.12. From the latter figure we could infer that loss of the function of the area striata in one cerebral hemisphere leads to loss of one half of the visual field in both eyes, so-called 'hemianopia' (Fig. 4.19).

The question now confronting us is one of the most important questions about spatial vision: is our directional localisation mirrored in detail in the anatomy and physiology of the brain? In other words: can we encounter the visual field, which summarizes the directions in our world in a polar co-ordinate system, in the brain?

This question is justified because it has long been known that the brain has a *somatotopic* organization, i.e., that fibres, nuclei and cortical areas are grouped in the same way as the body parts they represent. There are various somatotopic charts and these have different functions in the brain. The chart of the motor system (which has been established by electrical stimulation of non-anaesthetised patients undergoing a brain operation) is shown in Figure 6.9. The chart is out of proportion: the cortical representation of the hand is as large as that of the legs and trunk together. The somatosensory area lies just behind the motor area and is distorted in a similar way (Penfield & Rasmussen, 1952).

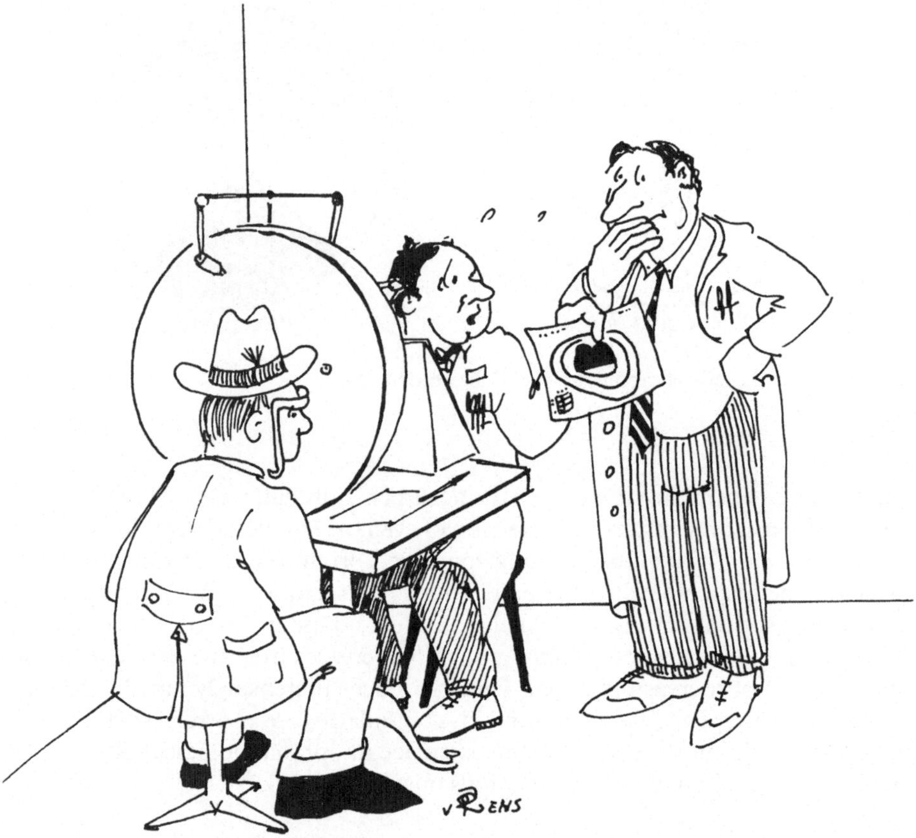

Fig. 6.8. Determination of the visual field. Problems with the projection perimeter (Van Rens).

It was at first uncertain whether the retinas had a precise topographical projection on the cerebral cortex. Certainty was only obtained in the First World War. The Irish neurologist Gordon Holmes analysed the effects of shot wounds in the back of the head. He compared the position of the wound with the patient's visual field defects. It appeared that the world was still represented upside-down in the cerebral cortex. Furthermore the representation is completely disproportional. The relatively small centre of the retina occupies more space in the cortex than the entire periphery. Figure 6.10 shows the visual fields of one of Holmes's patients together with the position of the wound. There is a small symmetrical visual field defect. It looks harmless, but it makes reading impossible because only the left half of each word can be seen.

CHARTING THE VISUAL FIELD IN THE AREA STRIATA

Modern studies have shown that the visual field is represented in the area striata strictly somatotopically but completely out of proportion. The area striata is the

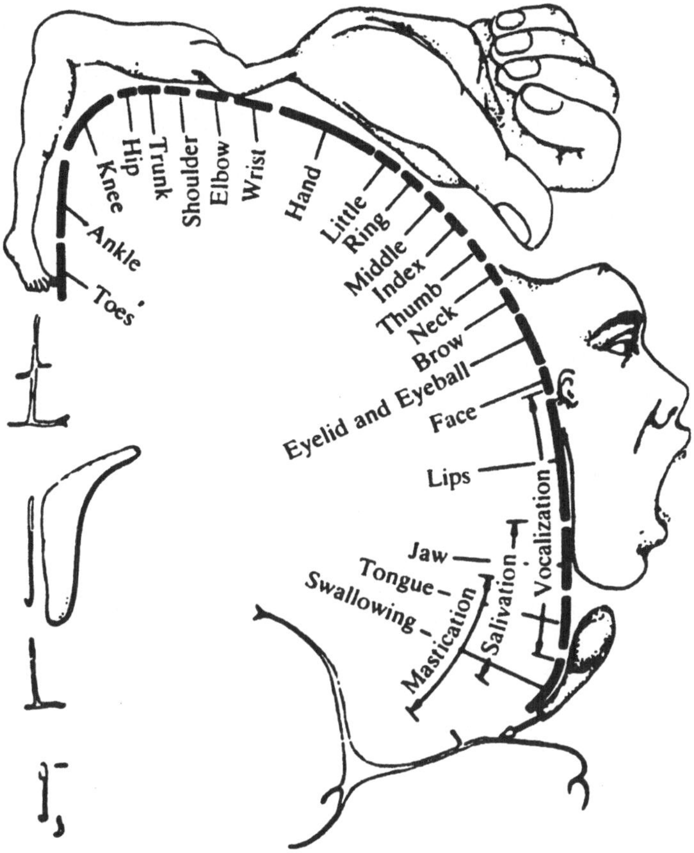

Fig. 6.9. Representation of the motor system of the body, drawn on a frontal section through the motor cortex of the brain (after Penfield & Rasmussen, 1952).

cortical area that, in neurophysiology, has been more extensively studied than any other area. Neurophysiologists have studied the electrical activity of cells on visual stimulation in anaesthetised and artificially paralysed animals. For this reason the information is mainly about the afferent role of the aria striata. The area striata contains approximately 500 million cells, which together process the information from two million optic fibres. In the retina the density of the ganglion cells at the centre is far greater than in the periphery. There are 100 million receptors in the retina, but only the cones at the centre of the retina have their own ganglion cells and thus their own optic fibres. In correspondence with this, 25% of the area striata is occupied with the processing of stimuli from the central retinal area with its diameter of 2 to 3 degrees. There is thus an enormous 'cortical magnification' of the foveal area. Figure 6.11 illustrates this strikingly.

A good image of directional vision in efferent innervations cannot be found in the area striata. That doesn't mean that the largest and most important visual area plays no part in the organization of eye movements; there is a massive projection of

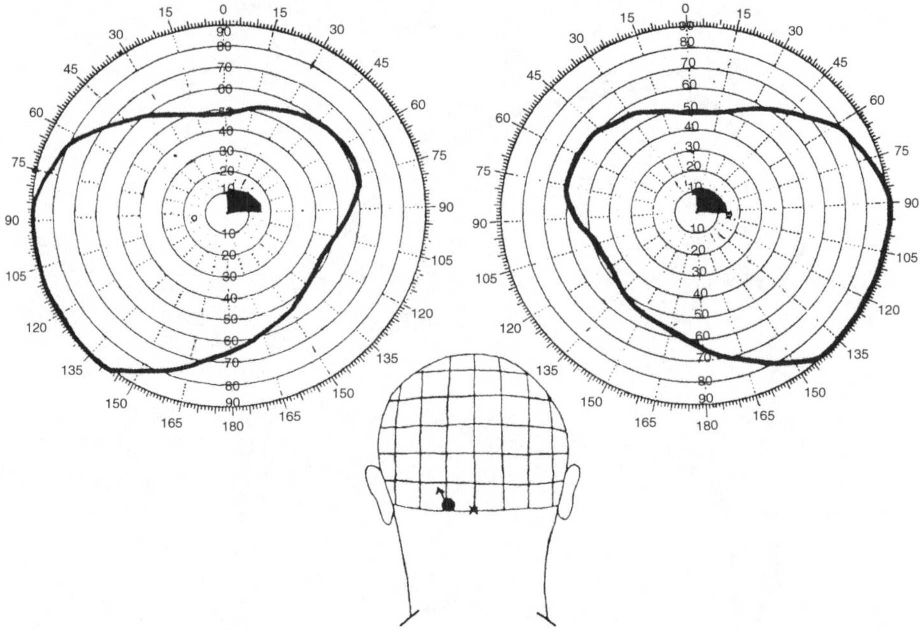

Fig. 6.10. Bilateral visual field defect due to a shot wound in the back of the head (Holmes, 1918).

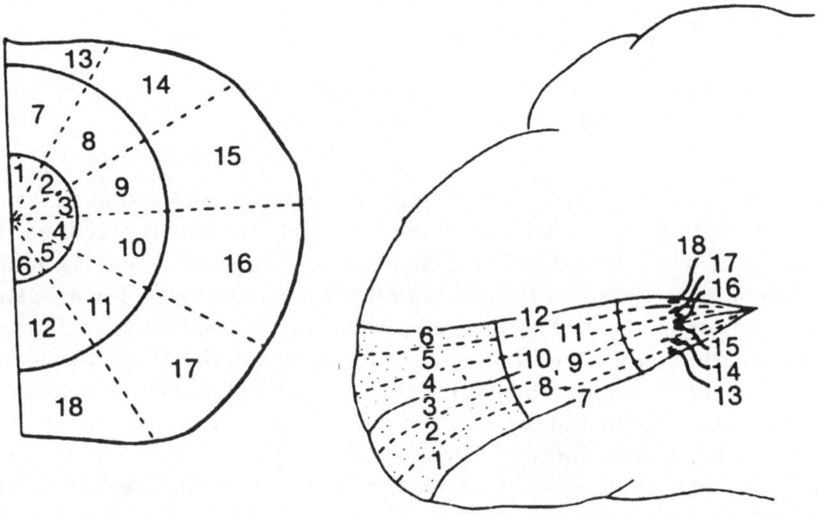

Fig. 6.11. Retinotopic representation in the striate area. The right homonymous half-field (left) and the left calcarine fissure of the striate area (right). The figure is based on the study of visual field defects in patients suffering from penetrating missile wounds to the brain (Teuber et al., 1960).

striatal fibres onto the superior colliculi (tract I in Fig. 4.16), the small nuclear area where ocular motor fibres from many visual areas converge. The superior colliculi also receive many fibres from other cortical areas that are important for directional vision (tracts II and III in Fig. 4.16).

What interests us in connection with directional vision is the *saccade*, the rapid eye movement which brings the image onto the fovea. This saccade is the motor effect of the stimulation of a peripheral retinal point: the direction in which we see an object in the subjective sense is translated into an equivalent physiological occurrence. Exactly how the precise equivalence is achieved is not yet fully known. The passage from retina to saccade takes place along many alternative routes where, not infrequently, the impulse in the fibres is in two directions.

The superior colliculi seem to be structures which, on the efferent side, are essentially involved in directional vision. Some preference is given to the central retina but the collicular magnifiation is nothing compared to that of the cortex. It is striking that there is a direct neural connection between the optic tract and the superior colliculus (Fig. 4.16). Not much imagination is needed to assume that this tract represents the strict and inflexible relationship between the position on the retina, on the one hand, and the definition of the saccade, qua direction and amplitude, on the other.

Naturally, the saccade is not the only, nor even the most important, motor effect of retinal stimulation. Grasping an object that is visible in a certain direction, is more important in the biological sense. But the neurophysiological implementation of this process is still largely unknown. So far we must content ourselves with the knowledge that the gaze movement is the first step in the sensorimotor process of directional vision.

PRECISION OF DIRECTIONAL VISION

THE PRECISION OF THE MOTOR SYSTEM

The saccade is a ballistic eye movement. Like a ball that has been thrown may reach its goal, or fall short of it, or go beyond it, so can the fovea land, or almost land, on the image of the object that was stimulating an eccentric retinal point. During the saccade no correction is possible, but small corrections afterwards do occur. The position of the eye then reached is incredibly precise. When we fixate a point of light, for instance for a minute, situated 25 degrees to the right of us, the *average* fixation remains accurate to one minute of arc[2]. That is 1:1000 precision! There is clearly a well-defined functional centre in the visual field (although this cannot be found in the fovea under the microscope).

But this precision only applies to the *average* fixation. In the short term, the eye in fixation is anything but still. The gaze has the tendency to drift away, first in one direction, then in the other, this being followed by a rapid movement that is usually centripetal (Fig. 6.12). This instability does not penetrate our consciousness and is therefore barely credible. But it is easy to be convinced by concentrating on the black spot in Figure 6.13 for half a minute and then looking at the white spot.

[2] Crone, 1984.

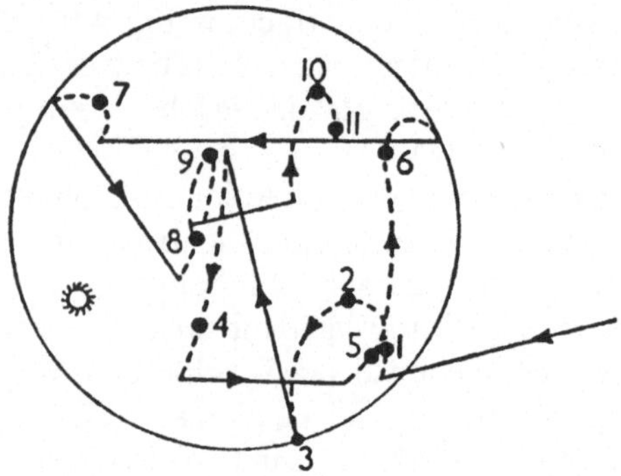

Fig. 6.12. The instability of the fixating eye. The image moves from one numbered dot to the next in 0.2 seconds. Diameter of large circle: 10 minutes of arc; small circle: distance between two cones (Ditchburn, 1955).

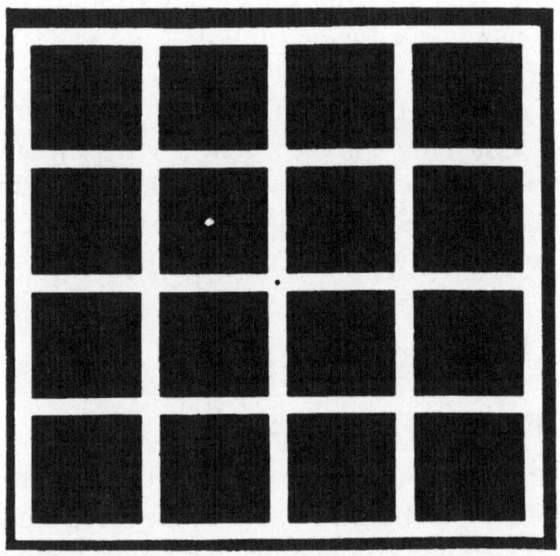

Fig. 6.13. Demonstration of unstable fixation. Carefully fixate the black dot for 30 seconds, then fixate the white dot. The black after-image of the white bars moves. Thus the image of the white dot moves over the retina (Verheyen, 1961).

A moving pattern of bars is seen as after-image. An after-image is stable relative to the retina. The fact that it is seen to move signifies that the fixation on the white spot is unstable.

It is not only looking in one direction, fixation, that works quite differently than we thought. Our conception of looking round in various directions is also completely wrong. We think that we can let our gaze glide over a scene like a video camera. We feel intuitively that it is better to compare the eye with a video camera than with a cine camera. The continuous image and the absence of a shutter system in the eye suggest a video camera. But in actual fact the reverse is true: snapshots are

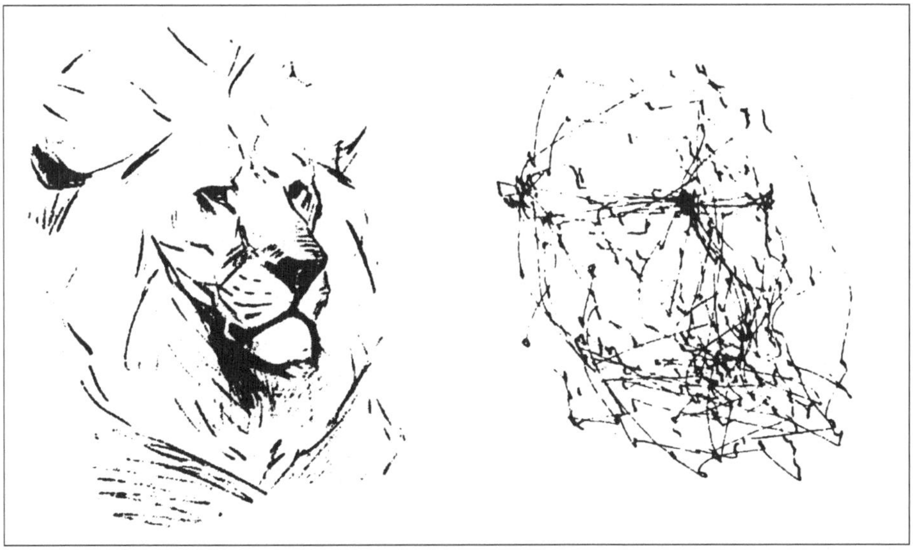

Fig. 6.14. Visual scanning. The drawing of a lion is studied for 2 minutes. Fixation jumps from one point to another, with preference for important contours. Perception takes place between two saccades. The registration was made by means of a ray of light reflected from a contact lens and a photographic plate (Yarbus, 1967).

being made all the time! When the eye seems to be gliding it is actually making jumps, saccades. Between two saccades the eye is still for a fraction of a second and a snapshot is taken. Figure 6.14, taken from the Russian research worker Yarbus, shows how the gaze jumps around the drawing of a lion for two minutes, with special attention for the most significant contours. When one is reading there is a similar succession of jerks. Between two saccades the eye sees a small number of letters.

THE SUBJECTIVE PRECISION OF DIRECTIONAL VISION

It is much more important for an organism to discover the difference between two impulses than to be informed about the absolute strength of one impulse. From the practical point of view the world doesn't change much when a cloud obscures the sun, despite the fact that the brightness markedly decreases and the colours change. On the other hand, when two surfaces are presented together, a difference in brightness of less than one percent and a colour difference of a few nanometres in the dominant wavelength can be easily recognized. This is also true for directional vision. In a dark room with fixated head, an attempt to localise *one* spot of light straight ahead in the median plane does not even achieve an accuracy of one degree, while the relative localisation of *two* vertical lines one above the other is at least 1000 times more accurate. When reading a slide rule with a vernier (Fig. 6.15) we achieve amazing accuracy. The 'vernier (nonius) acuity,' which in some countries

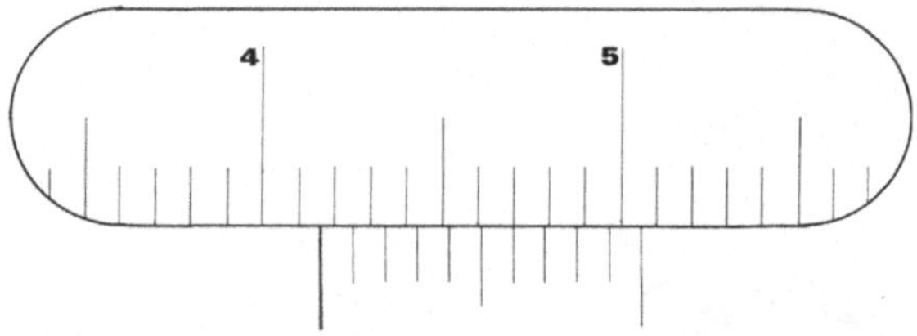

Fig. 6.15. The vernier of a slide-rule. Parts of the upper scale are read via a secondary scale with smaller units. The correct measurement is 4.16.

owes its name to a Portuguese maritime expert Petro Nunes (1492–1578) and in others to the French mathematician Pierre Vernier (1580–1636), is in favourable circumstances not more than a few seconds of arc. How this extreme sensitivity of our directional vision is possible is not yet completely understood. The explanation is made difficult by the extreme mobility of the eye. If directional vision is not to be misled by the vagaries of the eye, these will have to be reported to the visual centre. The eye muscles have a large number of stretch receptors which would be able to supply these reports.

VISUAL ACUITY, OPTICS AND CONTRAST

The minimum distance between two points which can just be distinguished (the *minimum separabile*, in Latin terms) is called the visual acuity. This distance is approximately one minute of arc. Hooke, Newton's great rival, knew that already. He could only distinguish double stars with the naked eye if they were separated by at least one minute of arc.

Testing visual acuity means testing the power of localisation. In the discussion of the noniusacuity it became clear that the eye is extremely sensitive to differences in visual direction; the threshold was only a few seconds of arc. Why is the threshold of visual acuity, i.e., the *minimum separabile*, so much higher? Two factors play a decisive role: limitation of the optical quality of the eye and limitation of our contrast sensitivity.

The visual acuity is of first importance in the assessment of sight. Almost every doctor has a letter chart in his surgery. The most common one is the more than hundred-year-old chart devised by Snellen (1862), at that time the first professor of ophthalmology in Utrecht. The letters are so designed that the details have an angular distance of one minute of arc when viewed at a distance of 6 metres. For special cases other charts may be needed (Fig. 6.16). The visual acuity, the measure of the distinguishing capacity for details, is a *psychophysical threshold measurement.* If someone with poor eyes can only distinguish two spots from a distance of 6 metres if they are 10 minutes of arc apart, the visual threshold is 10 minutes of arc. When assessing the senses people prefer to use terms of sensitivity rather than thresholds. The sensitivity is the reverse of the threshold. If a resolving power of 1 minute of arc is described as 'visual acuity = 1,' the above subject has a visual acuity of 1/10, the reverse of the threshold.

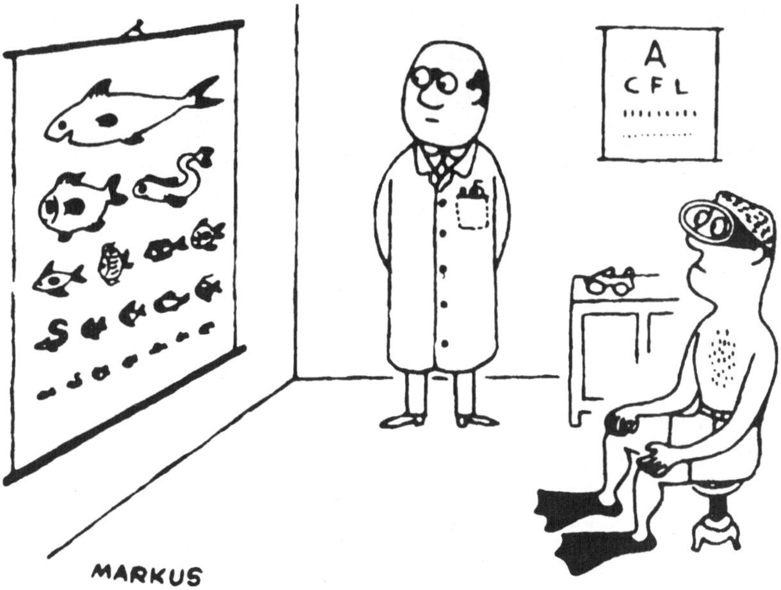

Fig. 6.16. Determination of the visual acuity.

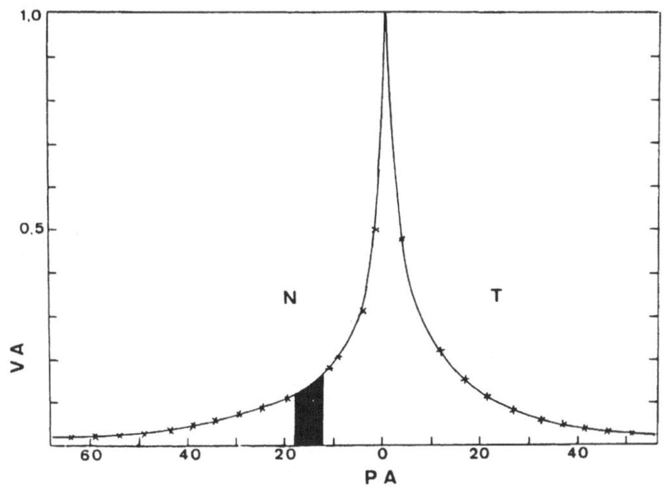

Fig. 6.17. Peripheral visual acuity, measured in the horizontal meridian. The black area corresponds with the papilla of the optic nerve. (PA) Perimetric angle at the retina; (VA) visual acuity; (N) nasal; (T) temporal (Wertheim, 1894).

The peripheral visual acuity

It is possible to determine the visual acuity of a normal subject when he is not looking directly at the letters. This produces the curve shown in Figure 6. 17, which was

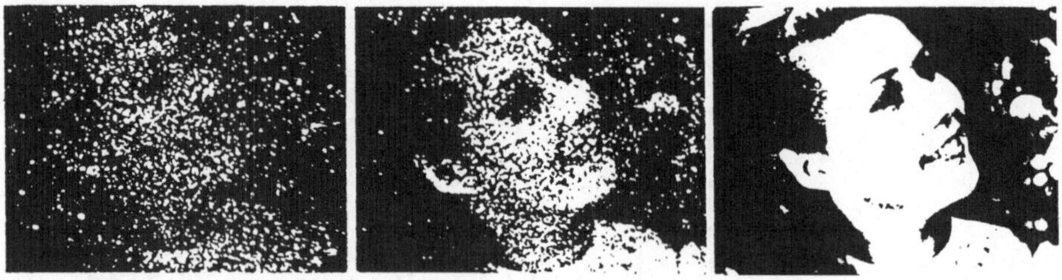

Fig. 6.18. The number of available quanta and the quality of an image (Rose, 1973). Left: thousand photons; middle: hundred thousand photons; right: thirty million photons.

obtained by Wertheim in 1894. There is a steep decline from centre to periphery, much steeper than would be expected from the quality of imaging. It shows more resemblance to Østerberg's cone curve, shown in Figure 4.9. The determination of the peripheral visual acuity is a difficult examination that is never carried out in practice. In the periphery points of light are much more easily recognized than letters; it is the method that is used for the determination of the visual field.

Vision in poor light

Two factors cause the decrease in visual acuity in poor light: the discontinuity of light and the switch from cone vision to rod vision. Since Einstein we know that light consists of quanta. If few quanta are available a good image cannot be formed on the retina (Fig. 6.18). But the resolving power of the retina also plays a role; it changes drastically in poor light. The light-sensitive rods come into action, but these work in groups. In addition, there are no rods in the fovea centralis. This leads to a marked decrease in visual acuity in poor light. A weak star disappears if one tries to look at it directly.

THE OPTICAL QUALITY

The optics of the eye are far less good than a good camera lens. The latter has only one fault—inescapable because of the diffraction of light—in the axial bundle: that a point is depicted as a diffraction circle, and this becomes larger as the lens opening (the diaphragm) becomes smaller.

The cornea and the lens which form the optic system of the eye, are living, nonhomogeneous tissues. One cannot expect the same perfection as that of a well-ground lens. As the pupil becomes larger the imperfection becomes more obvious. The visual acuity decreases. Figure 6.19 shows the results of a study of the imaging quality of the normal eye. A sharply defined line of light is presented to the eye; the retinal image of the line is reflected through the pupil onto a photographic cell which registers the spread of the light. The black circles are the measuring points. The thin line represents the theoretically attainable definition of the image on the grounds of diffraction. When the pupil has a diameter of 1.5 mm (or less) the definition of the image is mainly determined by diffraction. The best image is obtained

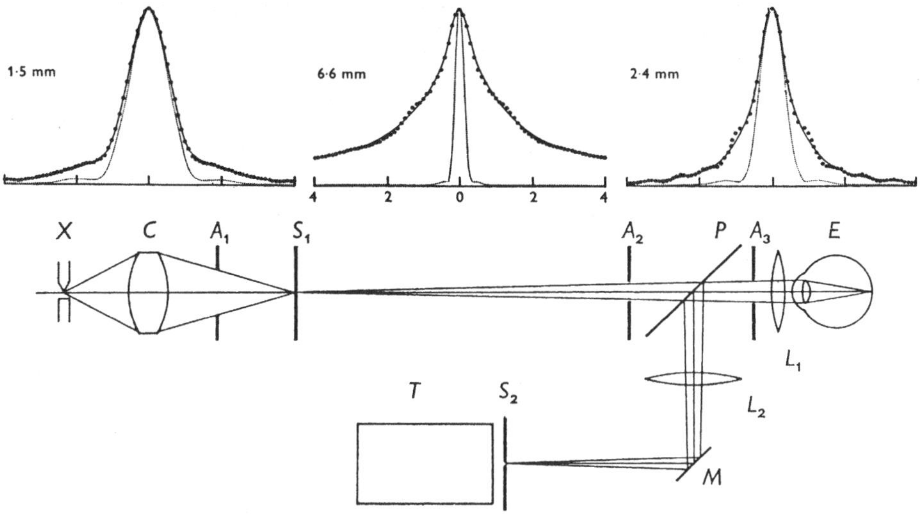

Fig. 6.19. The spread of a narrow line of light on the retina. Below: the line of light is imaged on the retina. The light reflected from the retina is reflected by a beam splitter P to the measuring apparatus. Above: vertical: intensity of light directed onto retina; horizontal: spread in minutes of arc. Optimum light distribution with 2.4 mm pupil. The thin line shows the scatter caused by diffraction when the optics are ideal (Campbell & Gubitsch, 1966).

with a 2.4 mm pupil, the measuring points then record the narrowest curve. With a larger pupil the definition becomes increasingly poor on account of optical problems.

CONTRAST

In the eye, with its poor optics, the definition of the image is to a large extent determined by its discernment of contrasts. When two spots are imaged next to each other on the retina, the distribution of light over the retina is as shown in Figure 6.20. If the eye is to see two separate spots, it must be able to distinguish the contrast between brightness A and brightness B. The limitation of the visual acuity imposed by the limitation of contrast sensitivity explains why the normal visual acuity is so far behind the vernier visual acuity.

VISUAL SYSTEMS ANALYSIS

For bioengineers and allied analytical minds, the determination of the visual acuity, as usually performed by the doctor, is an abomination (Fig. 6.16). The determination of the *minimum separabile* is confused by elements of form discrimination; the contrast offered is always maximum (black–white); the contours are always sharp. An attempt has been made to devise a general formula for the visual acuity, in which a standard stimulus on the (physical) input side could be varied in brightness, configuration (clarity of contours), contrast and visual angle; on the

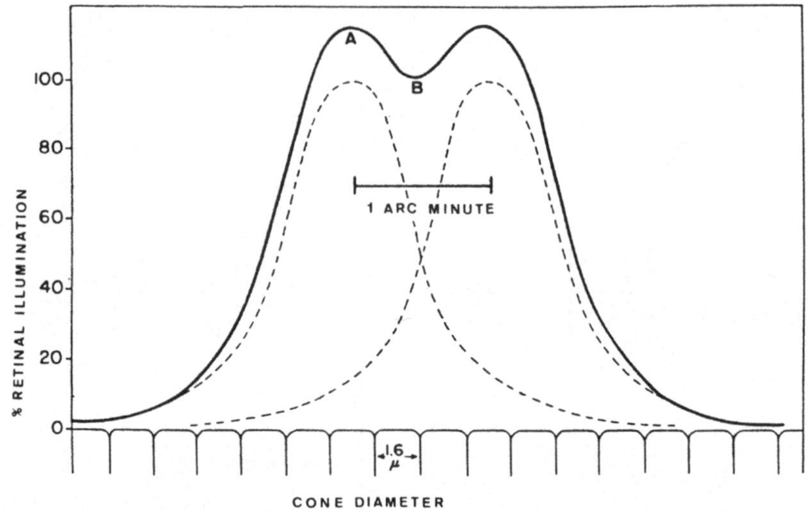

Fig. 6.20. Visual acuity is limited by contrast sensitivity. Two points separated by 1 minute of arc produce the light distribution on the retina shown by the dotted curves. The lights can be seen separately if the contrast between A and B can be distinguished.

(psychical) output side the threshold value of visibility would be measured, and by comparison of the input and output conclusions could be drawn about the intervening 'black box': the visual system. The *systems analysis* of spatial vision has led to important insights which, however, will not be considered in this book.

The inspiration for this process came in the fifties from a Dutch bioengineer, De Lange, who investigated a *temporal* visual threshold value, the critical fusion frequency (CFF). A flickering light stimulus is seen at a certain frequency as constant light. We are all aware of this phenomenon, in a film and fluorescent lighting. The frequency at which flicker fusion occurs depends on the configuration of the stimulus (wave-like or angled), the average illumination level and the contrast (depth of modulation) between the alternating light stimuli (Fig. 6.21). The maximum sensitivity to flicker is found to lie at a frequency of approximately 10 cycles per second. It appears that the visual system behaves (at least over a certain trajectory) as a linear system, whereby a sinusoidal (wave-like) input leads to a sinusoidal output, usually with the same frequency but quite often in a different phase. A non-sinusoidal input can, according to an old postulate by the French mathematician Fourier, always be resolved into a number of sinusoidal stimuli of different frequencies and phases (Fourier analysis). With the help of concepts derived from electrotechnology, De Lange was able to combine numerous empirical facts about the CFF under one heading.

A few years later Campbell and his co-workers applied systems analysis to *spatial* vision (Campbell & Robson, 1969). Input was sinusoidally varying gratings with different degrees of brightness, contrast and distance between the waves (Fig. 6.22) Output was the threshold value of the visibility of the gratings. The result was a curve

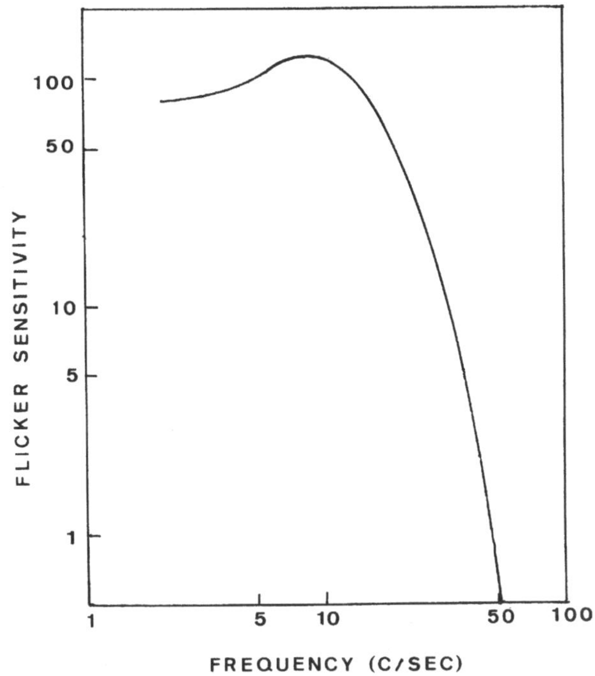

Fig. 6.21. Flicker sensitivity (reciprocal of modulation amplitude necessary to detect flicker at threshold), plotted as a function of temporal frequency (cycles per second), after De Lange (1952).

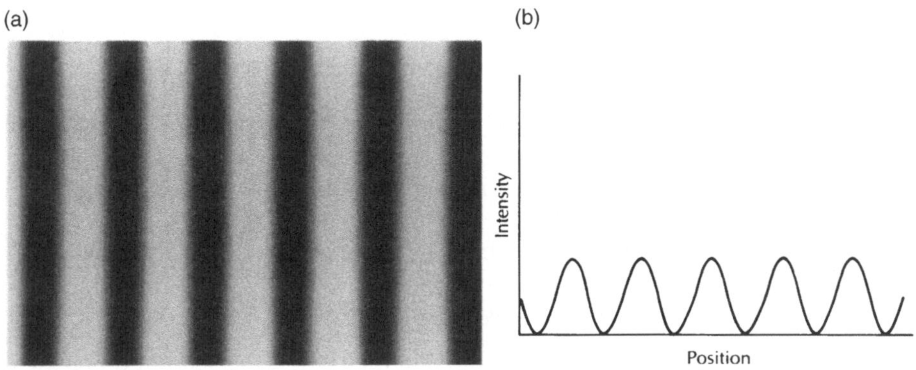

Fig. 6.22. A sine-wave grating.

as shown in Figure 6.23. The system was again found to be linear within certain limits and Fourier analysis could be applied. The terminology remained that of the alternating current technique: the angular distance between the sinusoidal contours was called 'spatial frequency,' 'high-frequency cut-off' (the end of the curve

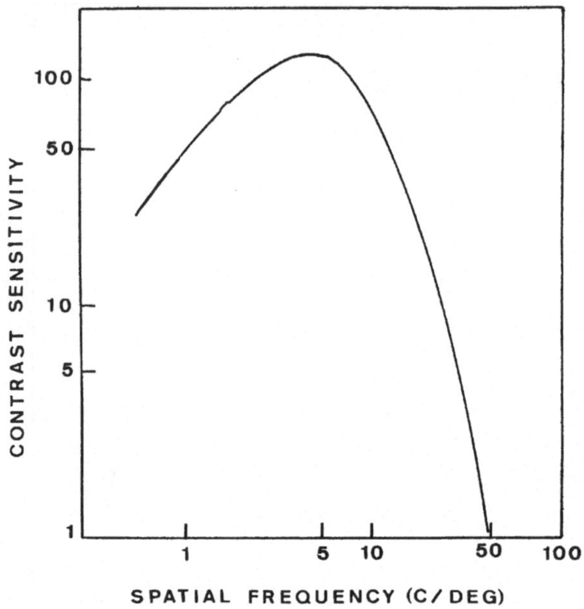

Fig. 6.23. Contrast sensitivity (reciprocal of contrast necessary to detect a sine-wave grating) plotted as a function of spatial frequency (cycles per degree), after DeValois (1990).

on the right) and 'low-frequency attenuation' (on the left) were named. Because negative light stimuli do not exist, sinusoidal stimuli were always superimposed on non-variable light, the 'direct-current component' of the stimulus. In short, the visual system was approached as an electronic 'filter' with specific properties.

Stimulation by sinusoidal gratings also has a disadvantage: the gratings are too wide for precise stimulation of the fovea. When a narrow 'wave-packet' is used instead, the position of the stimulus is more exact but the frequency is less precise. This is a situation which reminds one of the 'uncertainty principle' in quantum physics. There is also another disadvantage: for most visual scientists a spot of light is the simplest stimulus, but in the Fourier analysis it is one of the most complicated stimuli. A systems analyst looking up at the starry sky is demanding an almost impossible effort from his visual system.

THE NEUROPHYSIOLOGY OF THE VISUAL ACUITY

The description of the visual pathways in Chapter 4 and the section on cortical charting of directional vision have acquainted us with the various cerebral centres involved in the identification of direction and its subsequent motor effects. The description was a global sketch. It was as if one was walking in a large garden, where one knows the entrance and the exit and the paths by which they can be reached, but without noticing the plants and trees one passes on the way.

The neuro-anatomy and neurophysiology of the visual acuity have a quite different character. To continue with the example of the garden: one enters the garden and pays great attention to all the plants and trees in the first beds one comes to. One collects a wealth of information but does not penetrate further into the garden. The study of the visual acuity and other local details of vision has taken place in the first flowerbeds, the retina, LGN and area striata. The work has been performed on the microscopic level, especially by registering the electrical responses of individual cells and by refined methods of microscopic neuro-anatomy.

THE RETINA

The neurophysiological investigation of the visual acuity begins in the retina of an experimental animal. The animals react in different ways. Retinal ganglion cells which give a specific electrical reaction to movement are found in rabbits but not in apes. Important neurophysiological discoveries have been made in cats. Most of these will also be applicable to man. This applies to a much greater extent to experiments with apes. (This is particularly applicable to the neurophysiology of colour vision, because apes are the only mammals with colour vision comparable to that of man.)

Kuffler, an American neurophysiologist, performed experiments on anaesthetised cats (1953). He explored the retina with micro-electrodes and tapped the electrical responses of the—superficially situated—ganglion cells when the retina was stimulated with light. (These responses are extremely short action potentials, 'spikes,' all of the same height; the strength of the response is expressed by the *number* of action potentials per second.) At first Kuffler's results were disappointing: even when the retina was stimulated with a powerful ray of light very little happened. But when he began to stimulate the retina with a very narrow ray of light he got a lively response. Figure 6.24 shows the 'receptive field' of a ganglion cell that was put to the test by a micro-electrode.

The term 'receptive field' needs an explanation. Under the term 'receptive field' of a nerve cell in the visual system is understood that part of the visual field (or the retina) from which that nerve cell can be influenced by a light stimulus.

Many cells in the visual system have a certain resting activity. Influencing a cell can result in stimulation, excitation, through which the number of action potentials increases, or inhibition with the opposite effect. Whether excitation or inhibition occurs depends on the transmission substance in the synapse (see Fig. 4.10).

Figure 6.25 shows the behaviour of a cell which is stimulated when light falls on the centre of the receptive field. The ganglion cell becomes inhibited when the periphery of the receptive field is stimulated. When the periphery and the centre are stimulated together the responses are weak. The ganglion cell is clearly more interested in a small local contrast than in uniform illumination. A contour which is only half in the receptive field also stimulates more strongly than even illumination. Kuffler described both 'off centre' and 'on centre' ganglion cells.

Many ganglion cells are sensitive not only to differences in brightness between the centre and the periphery of the receptive field but also to differences in colour. In this book on spatial vision we need not spend time on this.

Some cells, the 'X cells,' have a very small receptive field and remain active as long as the light is on. Others have a large receptive field but react with short on

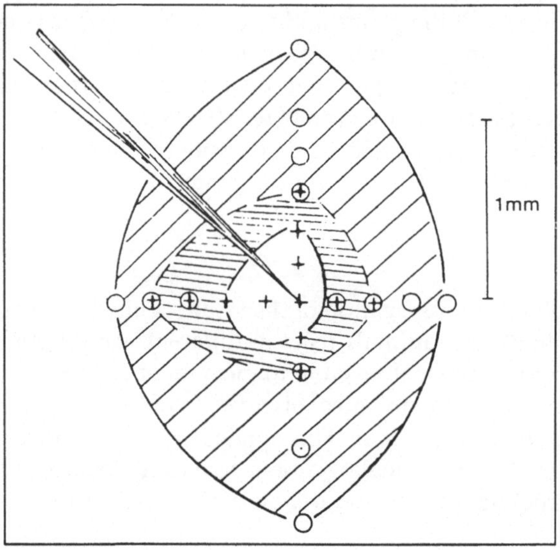

Fig. 6.24. The receptive field of a ganglion cell (Kuffler, 1953). A ganglion cell lies at the point of the electrode. Light at the centre of the field gives rise to impulses as the light goes on; at the periphery only when the light goes off. Between the centre and the periphery there is an intermediate area.

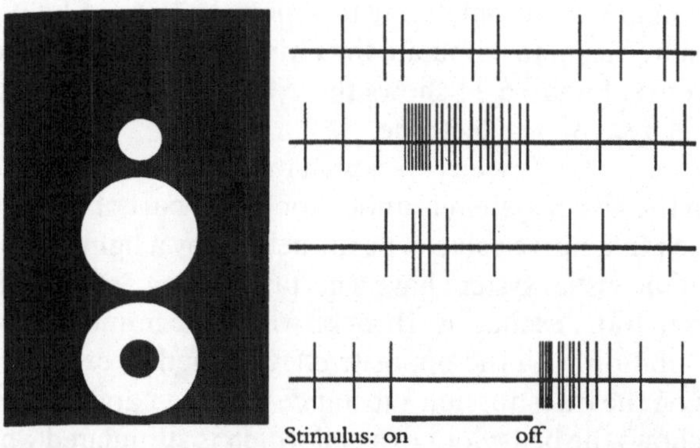

Fig. 6.25. Responses of an on-centre ganglion cell. To the left the stimuli are shown. In the resting state at the top, there is no stimulus, firing is slow and more or less random. The lower three records show responses to a small spot, a large spot covering the receptive-field centre and surround, and a ring covering the surround only (Hubel, 1988).

and out responses (the 'Ycells'). The X and Ycells can also be distinguished anatomically, and are then called beta- and alpha-cells. The former have their receptive fields mainly in the centre of the retina. They are attuned to the calm fixation of small details. The latter are designed to signal the rapid passage of events in the periphery of the visual field.

We here encounter the start of the neurophysiology of visual acuity: small receptive fields at the fovea, large fields in the periphery. Humans can distinguish two visual stimuli if they are separated from each other by a little less than one minute of arc. In the ape receptive fields have been found in the central retina which have a diameter of less than 2 minutes of arc.

THE LATERAL GENICULATE BODY

The fibres from the retinal ganglion cells pass the semidecussation in the chiasma and project onto the cells of the LGN (see Fig. 4.13). These small organs have four parvocellular layers and two magnocellular layers. The parvocellular layers contain cells which have small, circular receptive fields and are sensitive to colour. They synapse with the retinal beta-cells. The parvocellular laminae are thus the anatomical substratum of the visual acuity. The magnocellular elements have large receptive fields, are sensitive to movement but not to colour. The precise function of the LGN is not yet known, nor do we know why there are two sets of parvocellular laminae.

THE VISUAL CORTEX

In the visual cortex the processing of the retinal information is much more complicated than in the LGN. That is immediately apparent from a comparison of the number of neurones in the retina, the LGN and the area striata. The number of ganglion cells in the retina is estimated at about one million, in the LGN this number is almost doubled, but the area striata contains hundreds of millions of cells. The function of all these cells is still largely a mystery, but a corner of the veil was lifted in the sixties and later by Hubel and Wiesel. In 1958 the young neurophysiologist Hubel came to work in Kuffler's laboratory, with the intention of registering the action potentials of individual cells in the optic cortex when the eyes are stimulated by light. Such an experiment is not easy. A cat is anaesthetised and the head is clamped fast. The eyes are kept open and damp. Every movement of the anaesthetised animal is suppressed by the administration of a paralysing drug. Part of the brain is exposed and micro-electrodes are inserted into the optic cortex with the help of a micromanipulator. There is a screen in front of the animal's eyes onto which light stimuli are projected by a slide-projector. Electrical signals received—when the stimulus is positioned correctly—by the micro-electrodes are amplified and registered, and made audible as crackling in a loudspeaker.

The first results obtained by Hubel and Wiesel were disappointing. It was not surprising that diffuse illumination of the screen had no effect. That had already been demonstrated for the retina by Kuffler. But it was also difficult to activate cortical cells with a spot of light. Then something unexpected happened: when the slides were changed and the image of an edge travelled over the retina, tremendous crackling sometimes broke out. In this way an important discovery was made, which marked the start of a long series of discoveries in the field of the physiology of the visual cortex. A cell in the visual cortex was found to be most easily activated by moving a luminous line (of a given length and breadth) at a certain angle ('orientation') over the screen in the direction at right angles to the line. In this way the

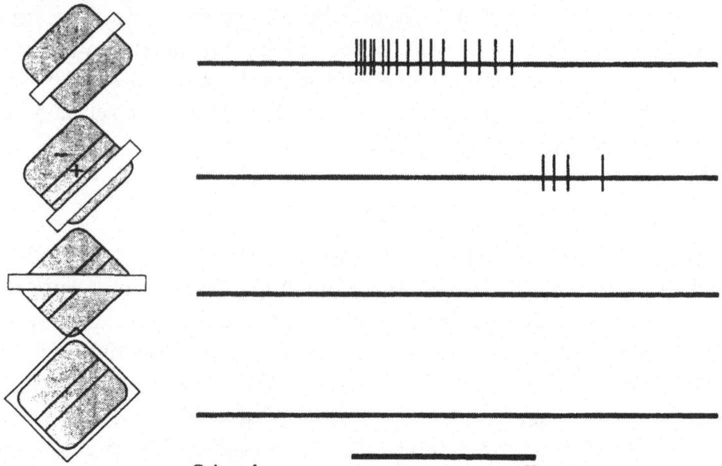

Fig. 6.26. The sensitivity of a neuron (with a central 'on' and a peripheral 'off' field) to the orientation of a line-shaped stimulus, presented in the period between 'on' and 'off' (after Hubel, 1988).

receptive fields of many cortical cells were registered. Various types of cells were found, each characterised by the properties of its receptive field. Most of the fields are elongated and have an excitation and an inhibition zone (Fig. 6.26); other cells have a small field and react to local contrasts, if these are presented at the right orientation. If an electrode is inserted perpendicular to the surface of the cortex, the cells that are sensitive to one orientation lie in one column of the primary visual cortex (Fig. 6.27). The visual cortex thus goes much further than the CGL where, in the size and antagonistic structure of the circular receptive fields, much was recognizable as the physiological substratum of the *minimum separabile.* In the cortex 'feature extraction' is much more complicated. I return to this extensively in the following chapters.

In the peristriate and higher areas we completely lose track of the visual acuity, but find it again at the end of the sensorimotor process of vision: the precision of average fixation (see p. 65) is at least one minute of arc, and is thus of the same order as the visual acuity (or perhaps even the nonius visual acuity).

VISUAL SYSTEMS ANALYSIS AND NEUROPHYSIOLOGY

The visual systems analysis has made its impression on the neurophysiology of the area striata. The cortical cells described in the last section could be characterized as 'bar detectors.' Another feature presents itself on stimulation with sinusoidal gratings: the same cells react—by presentation of a grating in the right place and at the same orientation—selectively to certain spatial frequencies, with marked loss of sensitivity when the frequency is higher or lower than the optimal frequency. The systems analysts think that certain cells are found—also on stimulation of

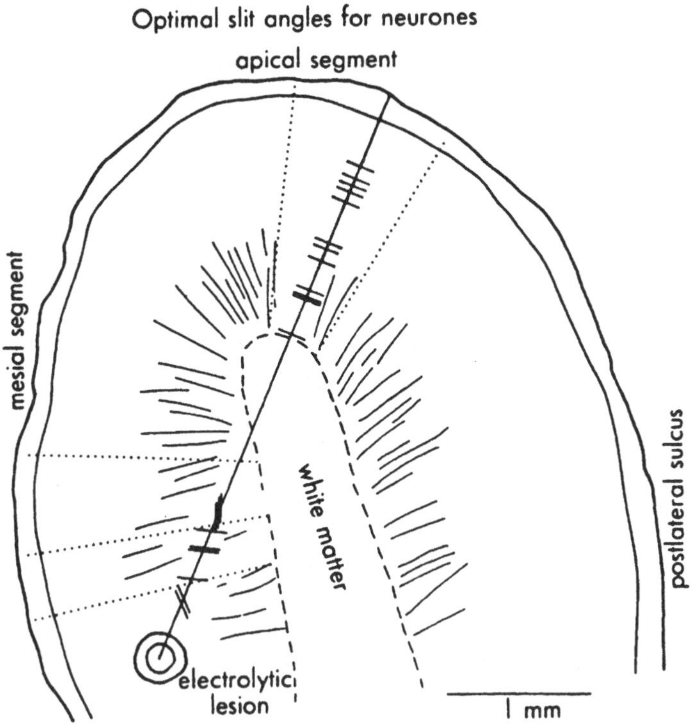

Fig. 6.27. Orientational responses of neurons in primary visual cortex of cat. When an electrode penetrates a cortical column the receptive fields of the cells encountered are sensitive to stimuli with the same orientation; further along, more columns are traversed and cells are found with differently orientated receptive fields. Finally an electrolytic lesion is made in order to be able to identify the path of the electrode in the specimen (Hubel & Wiesel, 1962).

the central retina—which are attuned to certain spatial frequencies. Following this train of thought, the spatial function of contrast sensitivity is the enveloping curve of many closely attuned channels which are selective for spatial frequency (Fig. 6.28).

THE PATHOLOGY OF DIRECTIONAL VISION

The pathology of directional vision, a subject that lies in the field of ophthalmology, neuro-ophthalmology and neurology, will hardly be considered here. That certainly applies to conditions which are associated with other sensory mechanisms, such as the vestibular system. In Chapter 4, a sketch was given of the various stations which the visual impulse passes on the way from the retina to eye movement. At all these spots a lesion may cause disturbance of spatial vision. Retinal conditions can disturb the regular organization of the receptors and lead to distortion of the visual image. Lesions between the retina and the area striata cause visual field defects. They form an inexhaustible source of neuro-ophthalmological diagnostics.

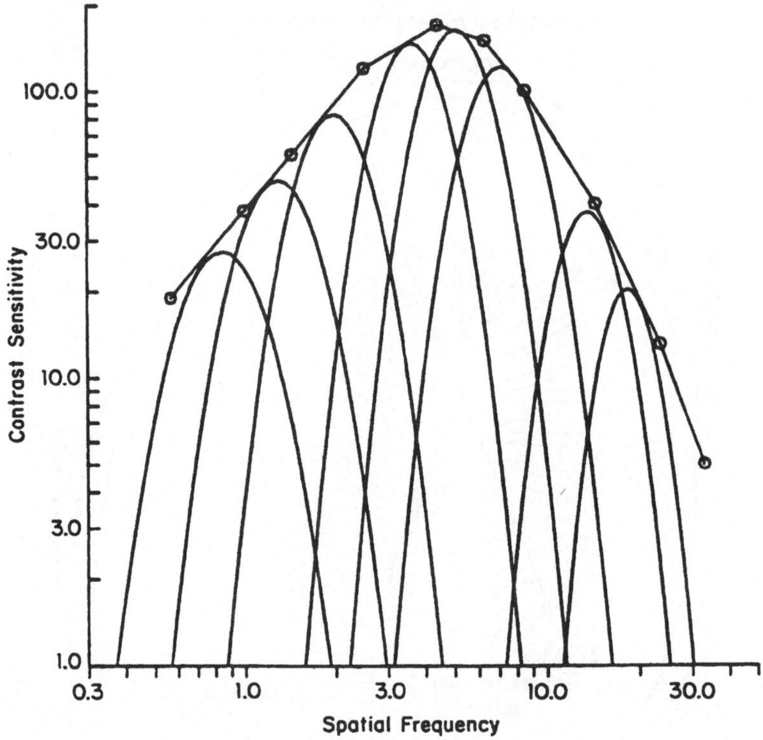

Fig. 6.28. The spatial contrast sensitivity function as the envelope of many more narrowly tuned spatial frequency selective channels (De Valois, 1990).

It is interesting that in some forms of cortical hemianopia directional vision is spared. Such patients can point to a light stimulus which is offered in the blind part of the visual field and is not consciously seen.[3] It is assumed that there is a sort of 'second visual system.' Optic fibres leave the optic tract before the LGN, traverse various subcortical structures and branch off to the prestratium. Apes whose areae striatae have been surgically removed still make a grab at cockroaches. In hamsters, after the removal of the primary visual centres, so much sight remains that only focal vision has been lost; rough visual orientation (ambient vision) still exists.[4]

Beyond the area striata visual field defects are no longer seen and disturbances of directional vision have a different character. Lesions of the parietal lobe often lead to disregard of the visual stimuli on one side (hemi-neglect). Patients with right-sided hemi-neglect draw a clock with all the hours on the left side of the clock face. The eye movements in the direction of the neglected half of the visual field may also be abnormal. Bilateral lesions of the parietal lobes lead to the loss of orientation.

[3] Stenvers, 1945.

[4] Trevarthen, 1968.

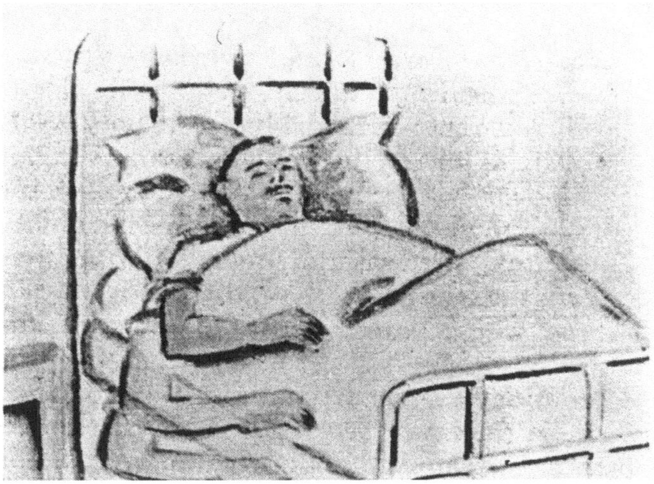

Fig. 6.29. Polyopia (Mooney et al., 1965).

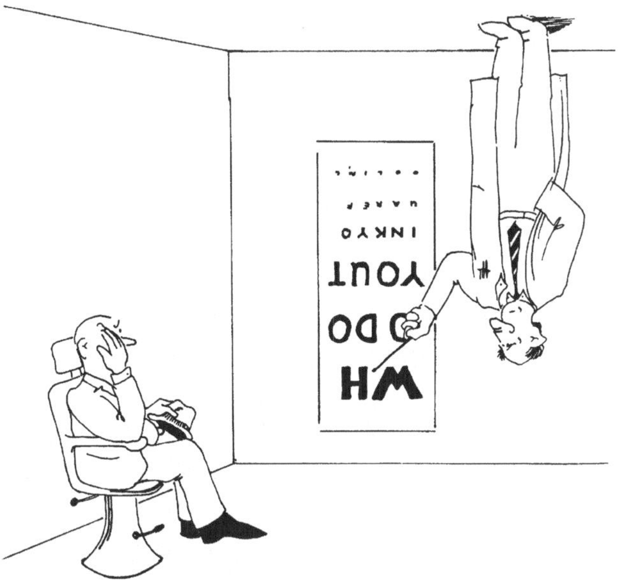

Fig. 6.30. Inverted vision (Van Rens).

Other anomalies of directional vision have also been described in cerebral conditions. For instance, objects can appear to be distorted (dysmorphopsia). Polyopia has also been described: the patient sees an object in several directions at the same time (Fig. 6.29). A rare and bizarre anomaly is upside-down vision[5] (Fig. 6.30).

[5] Klopp, 1951.

These are all conditions which are of great interest to the neurologist, but throw little light on the properties of spatial vision described in this chapter.

The most peripheral disturbance of directional vision on the efferent side is *past-pointing*. If a patient's right lateral rectus muscle is partially paralysed and he looks at an object on the right (with his left eye closed), the muscle must give an abnormally strong impulse to the right. The object therefore seems to lie further to the right than it actually is. A pointing finger (placed out of optic control by a screen) then points too far to the right.

Paralysis of the eye muscles gives rise to an important subjective symptom: double vision (diplopia). This is due to the fact that the directions of gaze are not parallel when looking in a certain direction.

7. Stereoscopic Perception of Depth[1]

A MODEL OF BINOCULAR VISION[2]

In the last paragraphs of Chapter 5, I have explained how the evolution of the visual system has led to binocular vision of depth. In primitive organisms such as the pike and the chameleon it had become clear that *convergence* was the principal cue to depth in those animals. But in birds and mammals there came a new cue to depth: *disparity* (p. 51). In mammals the semidecussation of the optic nerves brought *corresponding cortical points* (representing identical directions in space at infinity) into close proximity, making non-corresponding, disparate, points (representing a nearby object in space) easily detectable.

The functional results of the development sketched above cannot be deduced from Polyak's figure (Fig. 4.12), which shows only the macroscopic anatomy. Modern research into the microanatomy and microphysiology of the visual cortex has yielded important results, which, however, are not easy to visualize. Therefore, a simplified model of binocular vision is indispensable. It is pictured in Figures 7.1 and 7.2.

1. The complicated structure of the convoluted cortical visual area and the passage between the two hemispheres is replaced by a continuous line (BV, binocular vision), with the representation of the foveae (F) at the centre.
2. This continuous line BV symbolizes binocular vision, which has arisen through the meeting and cooperation of the cortical projections of the two retinas (CR and CL), or rather of the two horizontal retinal meridians of the retinas. As stated, this line of binocular vision is the result of the cooperation of retinal points, simultaneously stimulated by a distant visual object, which correspond in the visual cortex, i.e., are represented in close proximity to each other (in the diagram, *directly opposite each other* on both sides of the binocular line). The position of these two lines (the projection of the right retina above and the left below) is naturally completely arbitrary. In comparison with reality, this model is in many ways simplistic, but a diagram is essential when considering spatial vision.

[1] Julesz, 1971; Crone, 1973; Crone and Sanjoto Hardjowijoto, 1979; Hubel, 1988.
[2] Crone, 1969a, b.

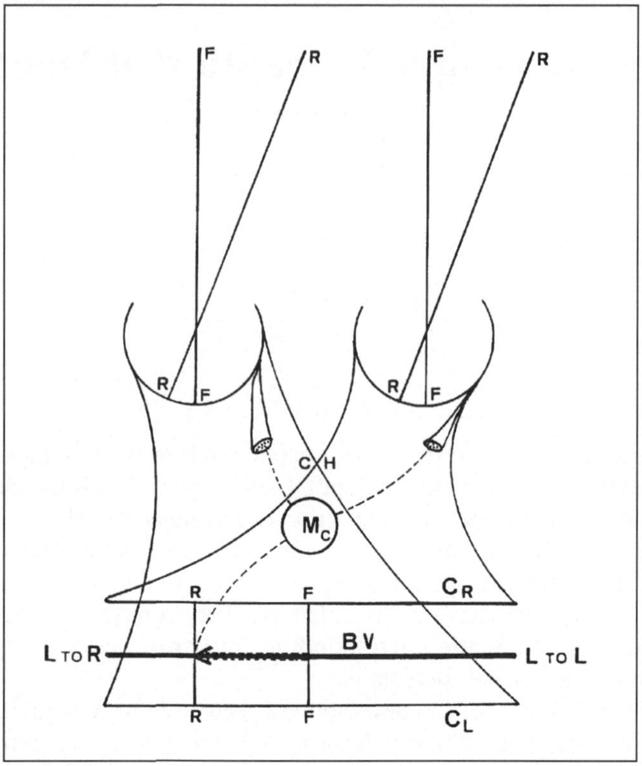

Fig. 7.1. A model of binocular vision (Crone, 1969). (BV) Line of binocular vision; C_R, C_L cortical representation of right, left retina; (F) far visual object straight ahead, foveae, cortical representation of foveae; (L to R, L to L) localization and saccade to the right, to the left; (M_C) motor centre in brainstem for conjugate eye movements; (R) far object situated to the right, its retinal projections, its cortical projections; broken arrow: path of motor impulse resulting in a saccade to the right that foveates R. For explanation see text.

3. In accordance with the basic principle of this book, which emphasizes the sensorimotor aspect of vision, this model tries to make a connection between retinal stimuli and movement. For this reason the projections of the retinas are strictly *retinotopic*: the distance between the cortical projection of a peripheral point in the retina and the fovea reflects the angular distance between the peripheral point and the fovea. Because the amplitude of a gaze movement also traverses the same angular distance, the amplitude of gaze movements (on monocular and binocular stimulation) can also be read from the diagram. The arrow in Figure 7.1 represents the impulse to a foveopetal saccade. This impulse is transmitted to the centre for conjugate eye movements, and from there to the eye muscles. Here again, I have resorted to a grave simplification: in reality the pathway from the area striata splits up and passes many intermediate stations (Fig. 4.17).

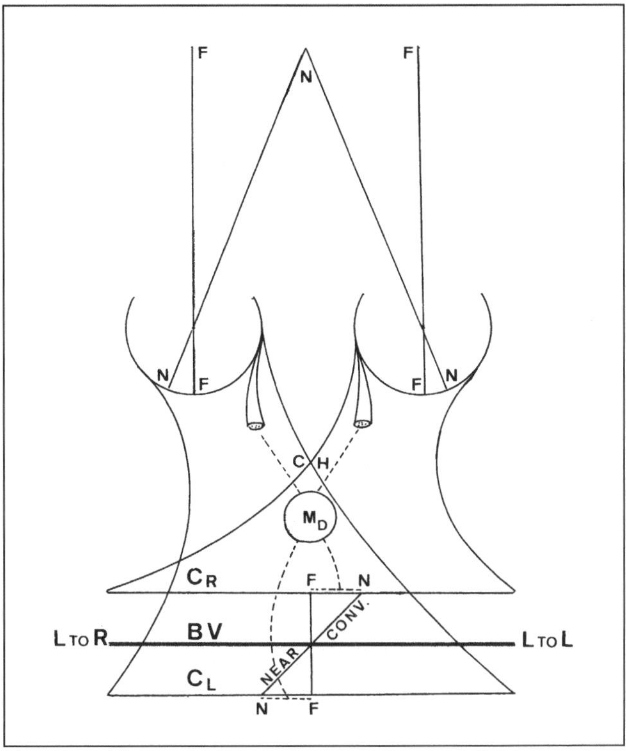

Fig. 7.2. Binocular perception of depth and convergence. Same diagram as Figure 7.1. (M_D) Motor centre in brainstem for disjunctive movements. The oblique line N–N denotes convergence and the localization 'near.' Broken line: path of motor impulse resulting in convergence. In order to fixate N, the right eye has to move to the left, and the left eye to the right. As the line N–N crosses the line of binocular vision at the zero point, point N is localized straight ahead.

But the mechanism of *disjunctive* eye movements can also be seen on the diagram. Let us assume (Fig. 7.2), that the eyes at rest are fixated on a distant object F. The central representations of the two foveae, situated directly opposite to each other, are stimulated by object F. All other distant points also stimulate representations in the same relative positions of 'corresponding' spatial points, which keep the eyes directed towards infinity. A closer object stimulates the retinas bitemporally. The central representations of the retinal points stimulated by object N lie *at an angle to each other* because of the bitemporal parallax, the (horizontal) 'disparity.' The oblique connection is thus a 'disparity detector.' Its obliquity is a measure of the proximity of object N. The disparity detector gives rise to an impulse towards movement of both eyes in the opposite direction, which impulse is transmitted to the centre for disjunctive eye movements, and from there (in the case of convergence) to the two medial rectus muscles. In their turn the points at infinity are now imaged on disparate (non-corresponding) retinal points. Figure 7.3 shows this for

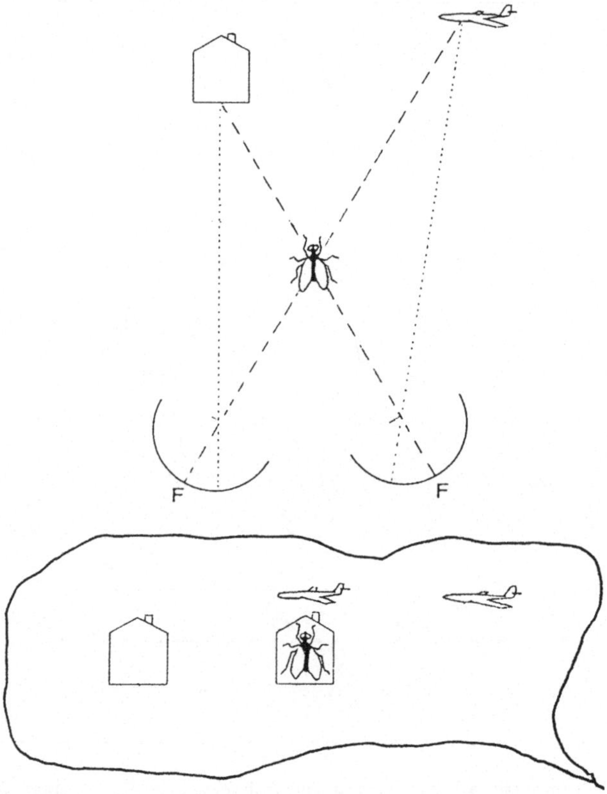

Fig. 7.3. Objects that are imaged on corresponding retinal areas are localized in the same direction.

the particular case where the disparate points are in line with the fixated near object. The distant points are then generally seen double, especially if attention is paid to the double image.

The model described above was designed to make the physiology of binocular vision more readily comprehensible. For this purpose it was necessary to simplify the area striata to such an extent that it has become an undistorted projection of the retinas. I emphasize that this retinotopic projection is in no way intended for the construction of a 'picture-in-the-head' which is more recognizable by the mind.

THE HISTORY OF BINOCULAR DEPTH PERCEPTION[3]

The fact that tasks which have to be performed close to the eyes can be carried out better with two eyes than with one, must have been known since time immemorial. But how binocular depth perception, stereoscopic vision, works was a problem for a long time.

[3] Wade, 1987, 1988; Crone, 1992.

Ptolemy (127–148), the famous Greek astronomer, had the first important ideas about depth perception. He was also an excellent experimental psychologist. For example, he painted sectors in various colours on a disc and observed the result when the disc was revolved. He also discovered 'physiological double vision.' For his examination he used two vertical rods placed one behind the other in the median plane. Ptolemy saw that the rod in front of the fixated rod was seen double and crossed and the rod behind was seen uncrossed. He also observed that the two rods seemed to be seen by an imaginary eye midway between the real eyes (the 'cyclopean eye' of the 19th century physiologists). If he had paused to consider that, between the two forms of double vision, there was a short trajectory close to the fixation point in which there were no double images but where, on the contrary, the difference in depth relative to the fixation point was exceptionally clear, it would have been Ptolemy and not Wheatstone (1600 years later) who was the discoverer of stereoscopic vision. Ptolemy knew nothing of image formation in the eye, but the process of stereoscopy could easily have been formulated in terms of psychological, phenomenal space.

Ptolemy also expressed an opinion on the position of the peripheral points which are seen at the same distance as the fixated object. This position was, according to him, the fronto-parallel plane which runs through the fixation point. (This is not exactly true: careful measurement of the position of the points on the horizontal meridian which appear to lie equally far from the fixation point, shows the position to be a curve with the observer at approximately the centre (see p. 95). But Ptolemy didn't have the instruments necessary to plot that curve.)

Ibn al-Haytham (1000), the great Arabian scholar known in the West as Alhazen, is the father of physiological optics. He tried to imagine how the rays coming from an object to the eye could produce an image of the object. He thought that must occur in the lens. The (upright) image was transported by the optic nerves to the (hollow) chiasma, where the images from the two eyes were combined into single binocular vision. In the discussion of depth perception Alhazen gave great weight to monocular criteria, such as the parallax of movement and apparent size, but also applies a binocular criterion: the consciousness of the convergent position of the eyes. Alhazen was the mentor of western optics specialists, like Roger Bacon and Vitello. Because Alhazen's 'Perspectiva' was their chief source of inspiration, they are still called the 'perspectivists.' Vitello (1270) made a diagram of binocular vision (Fig. 7.4).

Franciscus Aguilonius, rector of a Jesuit college in Antwerp, is the last of the perspectivists. He wrote a beautiful book, *Opticorum libri sex* (1613), about optics, which is illustrated by Rubens. Aguilonius, who is wrongly called the pioneer of binocular vision, took most of his material from Ptolemy and Alhazen. Figure 7.5 lets us see how well known it was that two eyes are important for the estimation of distance. To the delight of the cherubs an old scholar cannot judge the distance to the golden rod held in front of him when he has one eye shut. Figure 7.6 shows the scolar occupied with the investigation of the 'horopter.' The line through the fixation point in the horizontal plane and all peripheral points in the same plane are seen single on the frontoparallel plane. Like Ptolemy Aguilonius distinguishes crossed and uncrossed double images, *fallacii aspectus* (Fig. 7.7). Like Ptolemy

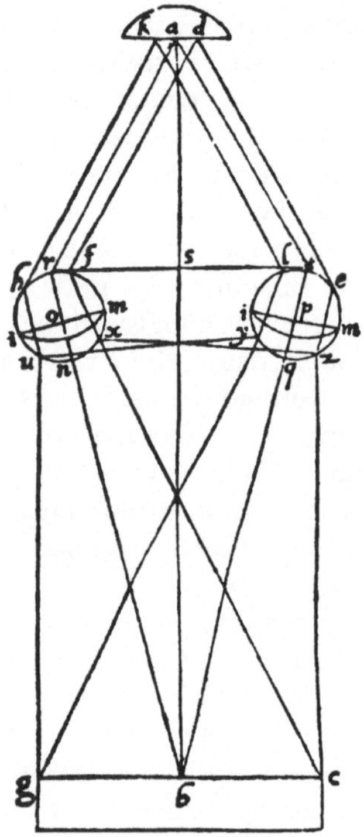

Fig. 7.4. An illustration from Vitello's Optics, Book III. The images from the two eyes are fused in the chiasma.

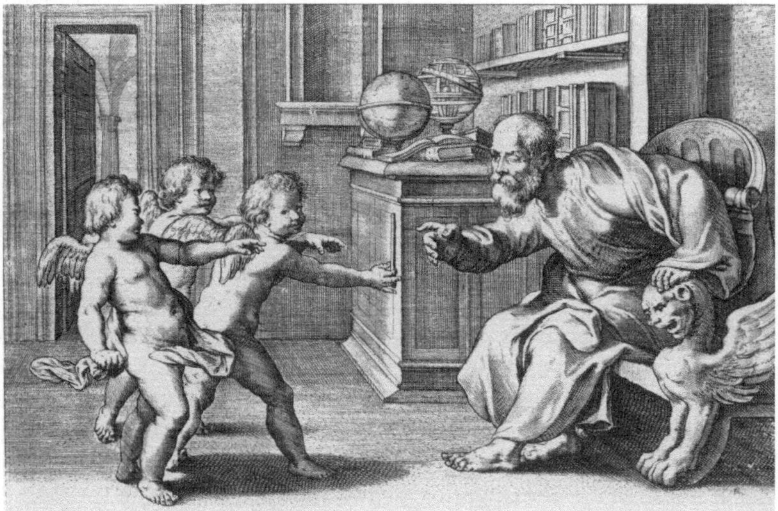

Fig. 7.5. The impossibility of depth discrimination with one eye (Aguilonius, *Opticorum lib. III*, 1613).

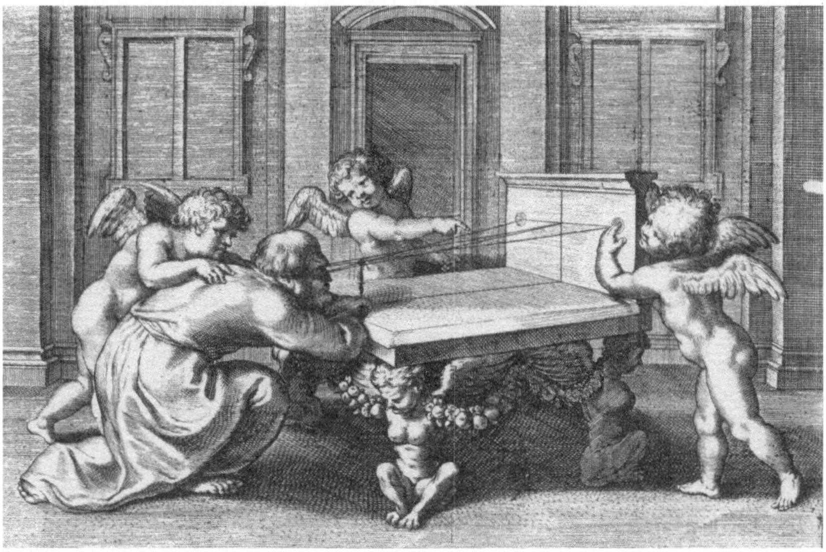

Fig. 7.6. The Horopter. When a point is fixated, peripheral points are seen single on the fronto-parallel plane (Aguilonius, 1613).

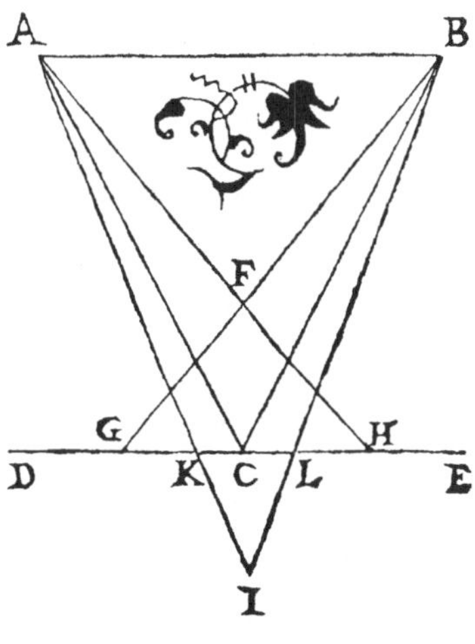

Fig. 7.7. The eyes A and B fixate C on the horopter plane. F and L are seen double (Aguilonius, 1613).

also, he localises the horopter in the fronto-parallel plane. He does not accept Alhazen's distance criterion (the sensation of convergence); if that was true the horopter would be a circle passing through both eyes and the fixation point. He illustrates that with a diagram (Fig. 7.8). If A and B are the eyes, the convergent angles ACB and ADB are equal.

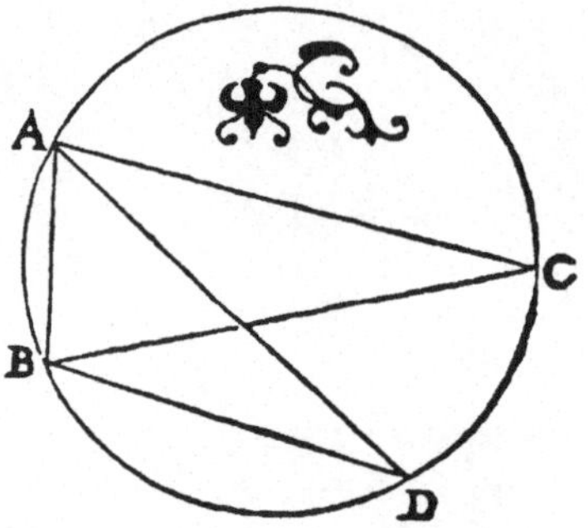

Fig. 7.8. Eyes A and B see all points on the circle, including C and D, at the same angle of convergence (Aguilonius, 1613).

Johannes Kepler, the Imperial Mathematician, had in the meantime (1604) discovered that the outside world is represented flat and upside-down on the retinas. This was a revolutionary discovery which did not make the solution of the problems of spatial vision any easier. On the contrary! How was it possible to see depth in two flat images? We now know the answer: there are small differences in the images on the two retinas which can be recognized. Of course Kepler also knew that the images in the right and left eyes were not completely identical, but he thought it improbable that anyone would be able to recognize depth from those minimal differences. His opinion was supported by a false observation made by Vesalius. The great Belgian anatomist had written that the optic nerves came very close to each other in the chiasma, but then continued on their way without crossing. In those circumstances, how could a subtle comparison of the retinal images in the head be possible? Kepler affiliated himself with Alhazen and concluded that the distance criterion was of motor nature: the convergence.

Descartes also accepted Vesalius' authoritative opinion (Fig. 4.19) and compared distant vision with the groping of a blind person with the help of two sticks (Fig. 7.9). Meanwhile, the idea was growing that the difference in perspective between the two retinal images might be recognized by the observer. That would mean that the two images would have to be, as it were, 'laid on top of each other' in order to be able to discover the extremely small differences. *Christiaan Huygens* introduced the term 'corresponding retinal points' in this connection. He meant the retinal points which, in each eye during binocular vision, were stimulated by the same visual object. The French physicist *Rohault*, who was still a follower of Vesalius, conceived a bold construction, shown in Figure 7.10, of a half crossing of the optic fibres in the brain. (This half crossing behind the chiasma does really exist (Fig. 5.10), not in man but in birds.)

Isaac Newton (1704) spoke the redeeming word in his *Opticks* shortly afterwards: half of the fibres cross in the chiasma. The first illustration of the half crossing (Fig. 7.11) derives from the famous and infamous travelling eye doctor Taylor, who in a later chapter will receive more attention.

Now the chance to explain binocular depth perception was there for the grasping: the brain must be able to detect disparities and thus experience depth sensations.

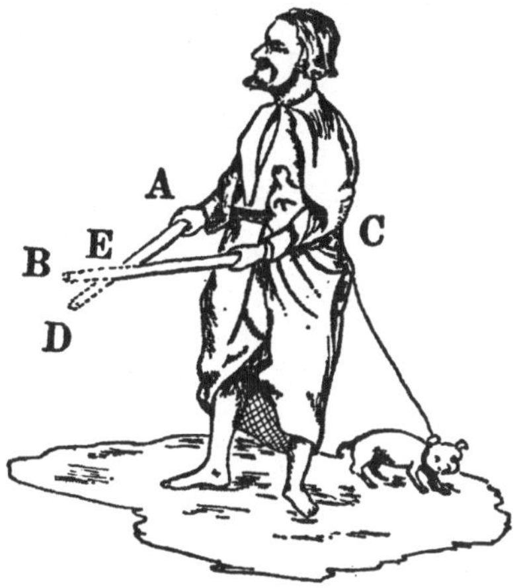

Fig. 7.9. According to Descartes we use our convergence to stimulate distance, in the same way as a blind man uses two sticks.

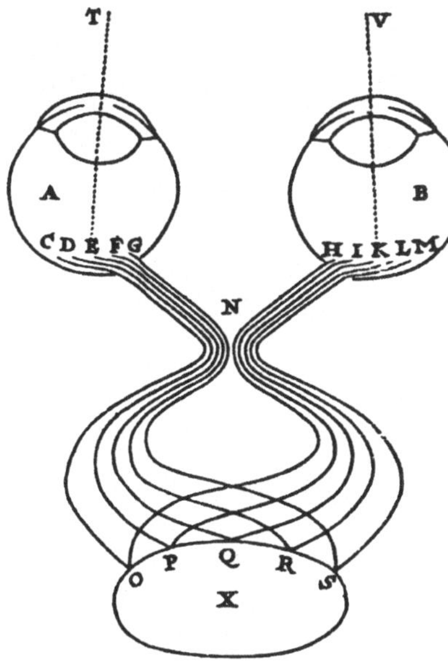

Fig. 7.10. The fusion of binocular images by a semidecussation of the optic fibres in the brain (Rohault, 1672).

But the chance was not grasped. The English empiricists like Locke and Berkeley, supported by the Cheselden case, had denied the eyes the potential to see depth (p. 22). An exceptional outsider had first to appear, who could demonstrate that binocular depth perception worked.

Charles Wheatstone, inventor and physicist, demonstrated in 1838 that with two flat plates one was able to see depth. Euclid had already said that the bottom of a vase

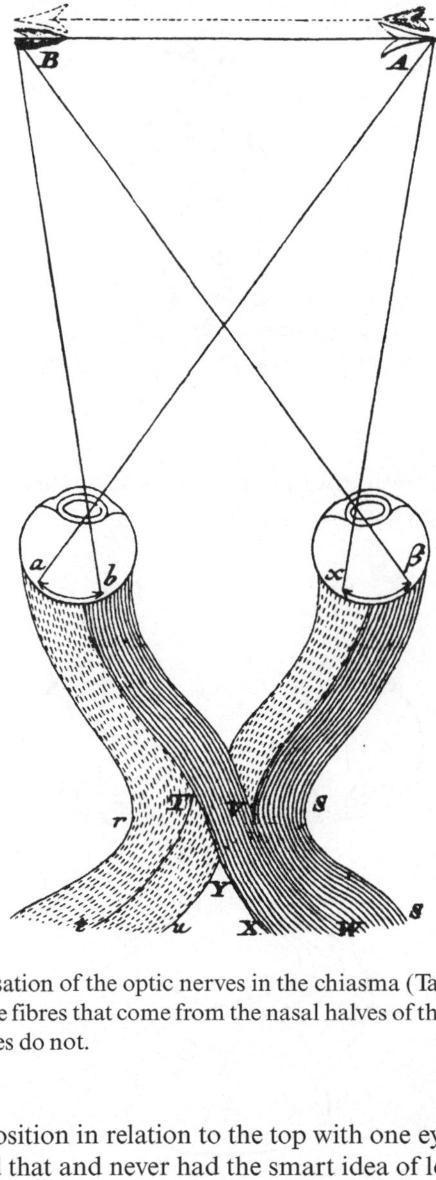

Fig. 7.11. Semidecussation of the optic nerves in the chiasma (Taylor, 1750). According to Newton's hypothesis the fibres that come from the nasal halves of the retinas cross, but those from the temporal halves do not.

took up a different position in relation to the top with one eye than with the other. He had just accepted that and never had the smart idea of looking to see whether two flat stereo-plates had the same depth effect. Wheatstone did just that, and built his stereoscope for the purpose (Fig. 7.12). In his very first publication on stereoscopy he penetrated to the heart of the problem: *depth is seen with the help of non-corresponding retinal points.* He was completely right, although the leap from the phenomena to the physiology (the retina) was not really necessary. What Wheatstone had discovered lies in the field of experimental psychology. It would have been sufficient to declare that single vision with depth perception is based on the binocular combination of spatial points with different monocular directions. Wheatstone confirmed with his discovery the autonomous nature of vision, independent of

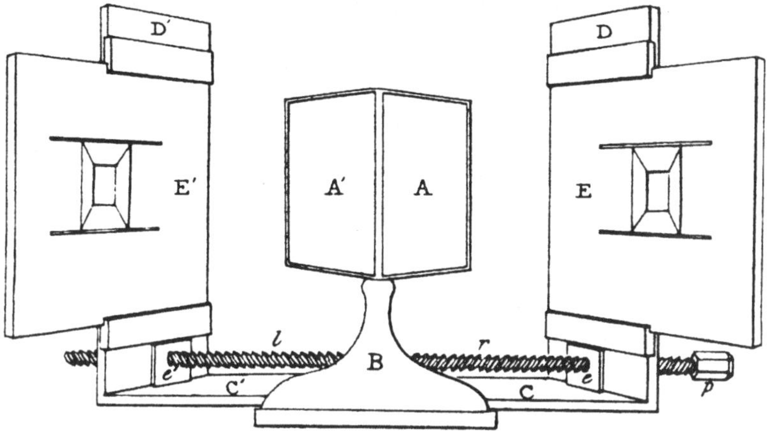

Fig. 7.12. Wheatstone's stereoscope (1838). The right eye sees plate E reflected in mirror A. The left eye sees E′ via A′. The two images are combined into one.

touch, and thus, without knowing it, sounded the knell of the empiricist theory. Wheatstone himself supported the empiricist view that depth perception had to be learned. That was later found to be untrue.

Wheatstone worked with laboriously drawn stereograms and cumbersome apparatus. His discovery therefore only drew the attention of scholars. But soon this changed. The Scottish physicist Brewster made a small, simple and inexpensive stereoscope in which Wheatstone's mirrors were replaced by prisms. Furthermore, only a few years later photography was invented. Soon people began to make stereo-cameras (with two lenses next to each other at eye distance). In 1851, at the World Exhibition in London, the French showed a series of beautiful stereo-daguerreotypes. Stereoscopy became so popular that half a million stereoscopes were sold in the next five years.

SOME PSYCHO-PHYSIOLOGICAL ASPECTS OF STEREOPSIS

PHYSIOLOGICAL DOUBLE VISION: THE RANGE OF THE OBLIQUE CONNECTIONS

Someone who looks at his finger and at the same time pays attention to a distant object, discovers that he sees that object double. This is called physiological double vision (diplopia); it was well known to Ptolemy. It should be distinguished from pathological double vision, which may occur when eye muscles are paralysed. When the right eye is closed, the right image disappears and vice versa. This is called uncrossed double vision or *homonymous diplopia*. If the subject looks at the distant object, he sees the finger double. If he closes his right eye the left finger disappears and vice versa: this is crossed double vision or *heteronymous diplopia*.

When an object is just behind or just in front of the fixated object, the difference in depth is perceived without seeing double. The depth which can be bridged without double vision is determined by the range of the oblique binocular connections.

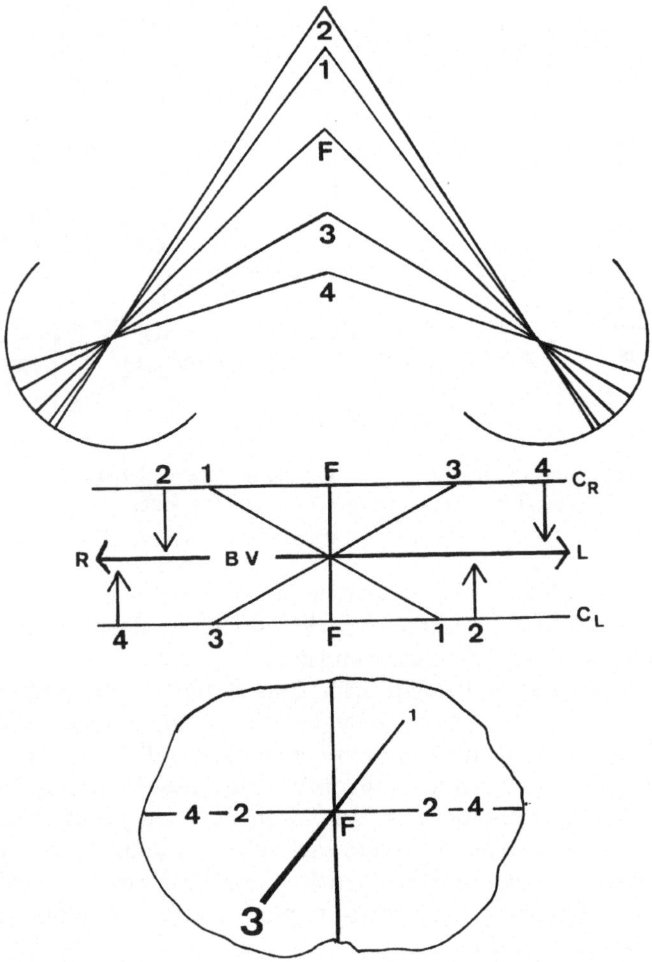

Fig. 7.13. The diplopia threshold. Middle: an oblique binocular connection is possible between the points 1 and 3. Bottom: Stereopsis in the primary direction of vision from points 1 to 3. Diplopia for points 2 (uncrossed) and 4 (crossed). For other symbols see Fig. 7.2.

In Figure 7.13 a number of points are lying one behind the other in the median plane. Point F is being fixated. The range of the oblique connections lies between points 1 and 3. This is the diplopia-free zone in the horizontal meridian.

Vertically disparate points can also be seen as one (although to a lesser extent and without the depth effect). This is practical because near objects seen to the right above the horizontal meridian, reach the right eye at a greater vertical angle than the left eye.

The diplopia-free zone is at the centre of the retina; in a laboratory test intended to detect the earliest possible trace of double vision, it is found to be small, measuring horizontally 10 minutes of arc and vertically even less. In tests which more

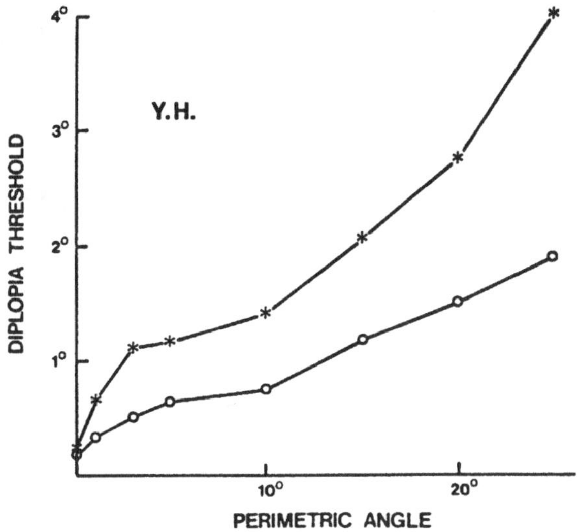

Fig. 7.14. Diplopia thresholds, vertical (circles) and horizontal (stars), as functions of the perimetric angle (Crone & Leuridan, 1973).

closely resemble natural conditions, the horizontal measurement of the diplopia-free zone may increase to more than 2 degrees. In the periphery the diplopia thresholds are higher, increasing more or less in step with the perimetric angle. This also applies to the vertical diplopia threshold. The curves in Figure 7.14 were obtained by noting how far two flashes had to be separated from each other (horizontally or vertically) to be seen as double. The diplopia zones in the periphery are also usually elliptical, as appears from the fact that the vertical diplopia thresholds in Figure 7.14 are lower than the horizontal ones.

THE HOROPTER

We return once again to the diagram in Figure 7.1 and the problem of binocular corresponding points. According to 7.1 binocular corresponding cortical elements are the projection of points which are seen by both eyes in the same direction. When both foveae are fixated on a distant point, it seems rather unnecessary to prove that peripheral objects are also seen in the same direction. If one is nevertheless determined to do this, one can go to work as follows: a distant traffic light, with a red and a green light one above the other, is fixated. Spectacles are put on with a red right glass and a green left glass, then one only sees the red light with the right eye and the green light with the left eye. If the red and green lights are exactly one above the other, even when looked at from the side, then they are seen in the same direction and thus stimulate corresponding cortical elements. The identity of the visual directions can be more precisely examined by using linear red and green lights one above the other: the 'vernier method.'

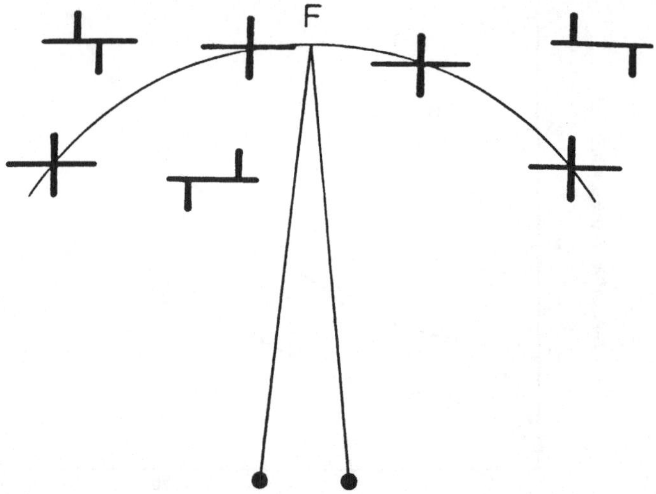

Fig. 7.15. The longitudinal horopter. Both eyes are focussed on F. The points at which the nonius lines are seen as one continuous line are all at approximately the same distance from the observer.

Let us now pass on to Figure 7.2. After the eyes have converged to point N, the two corresponding points NR and NL are opposite each other, are non-disparate and maintain the convergence impulse. In the diagram, and in the meridional spatial plane, where do all the other points lie which are seen by both eyes at the same depth? Intuitively one will say that they must lie just as far from the egocentre as the fixation point. Vernier examination shows that this is more or less the case. The empirical longitudinal (in the horizontal plane) horopter is the equidistant horopter, as appears from Figure 7.15.

But there is one problem: while there is an exact correlation between the directional vision and the size of the saccade, that is not true for peripheral near vision and convergence. *The points which give rise to the same convergence do not lie on the horopter*, but on a circle running through the eyes and the fixation point (Fig. 7.16, and 7.8). Somewhere in the visual system a correction must have taken place, with the result that binocularly corresponding points are not the projection of points that give rise to the same motor impulses. An enormous amount of rather uninspired academic literature has not led to a decision on how this process works.

THE LIMITS OF DEPTH PERCEPTION

ESTIMATION OF ABSOLUTE STEREOSCOPIC DEPTH

As was discussed for directional vision, in binocular depth perception the perception of *relative* depth (of one object in relation to another) is more important than the estimation of the *absolute* distance from the visual egocentre. In fact, this estimation for distant objects in an empty space is impossible.

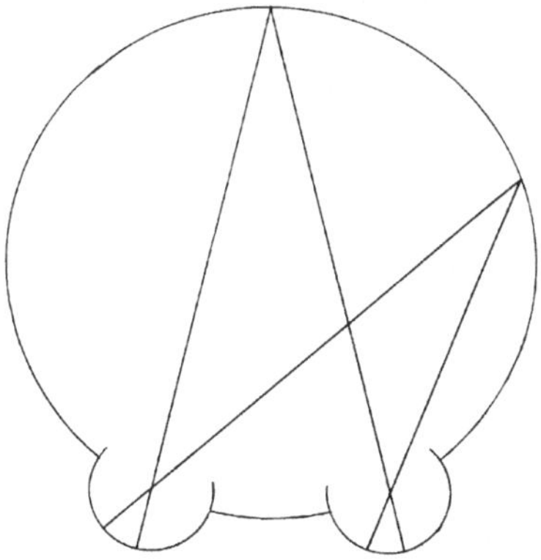

Fig. 7.16. The 'geometrical' horopter. The eyes see all the points on the circle at the same angle of convergence.

When an object is nearby there are ways of estimating the absolute distance: the convergence and the associated accommodation. The disparity-driven convergence has a high objective precision, but the information that it supplies for the estimation of absolute depth is imprecise (but better than that provided by the accommodation). A simple test shows how convergence contributes to the estimation of depth: one looks at an object, then puts on spectacles with base-out prisms (which force the eyes to stronger convergence), the object then appears to be closer and thus smaller. Base-in prisms have the opposite effect.

ESTIMATION OF RELATIVE STEREOSCOPIC DEPTH

Static stereopsis

The sensitivity of the human binocular depth perception is extremely great. Even a disparity of a few seconds of arc is recognized as depth. When one of a pair of rods is standing a couple of millimetres in front of the other, this can be seen in favourable circumstances at a distance of 100 metres. It is not surprising that the stereo-threshold is scarcely higher than the threshold for directional perception (the vernier visual acuity), in view of the intimate relationship that the binocularly corresponding points in the visual centre have with each other.

Disparity is expressed as an *angular* measure (angle 2 minus angle 1, see Fig. 7.17). *Linear* depth thresholds vary greatly with distance. The following table is easy to remember:

Distance:	20 cm	Threshold:	1/20 mm
	1 m		1 mm
	10 m		10 cm
	100 m		10 m

The discernment of depth, expressed as a linear measure, therefore becomes increasingly imprecise as the distance becomes greater. If we regard the threshold

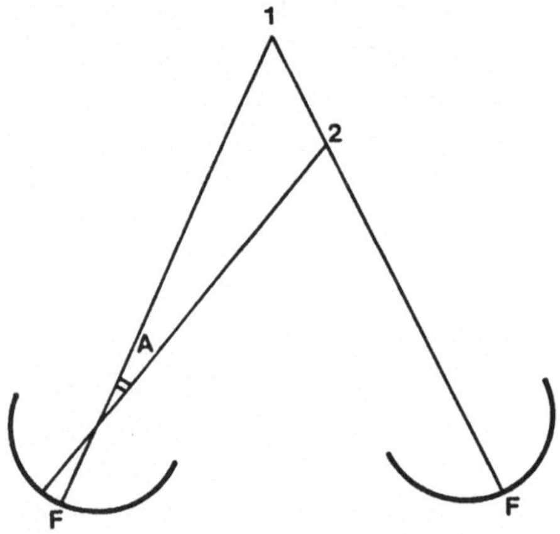

Fig. 7.17. Stereopsis. A: angle of disparity.

values of depth perception as the building blocks of stereoscopic space, then space is far from Euclidean.

Stereoscopic vision also has a lower limit. When the disparity is too great a double image is seen and the depth effect disappears. Whereas the upper threshold of stereoscopic sensitivity can be precisely measured, the lower threshold is rather vague. When double vision appears, the depth effect doesn't disappear immediately. There is an area in which diplopia and effective depth perception exist together. In the simplified diagram in Figure 7.13 this was not shown.

Kinetic stereopsis

The above applies to 'static stereopsis.' 'Kinetic stereopsis' also exists, to which other rules apply. In anticipation of what will be said in a later chapter about the perception of movement, kinetic stereopsis must now be considered.

While the static stereopsis described so far is a perfect aid to fine handicrafts, kinetic stereopsis has a quite different purpose: to avoid a stone that is flying towards your face or to catch a ball which is approaching your hand. Vision can then be content with a fairly rough detection of disparity that does not exclude diplopia and is accompanied by equally inexact convergence, as long as a rapid motor reaction is produced. As will be shown in a later section, kinetic stereopsis is a faculty *sui generis* with its own neurophysiological mechanism. Another phenomenon also helps us to perceive a rapidly approaching object: the object becomes larger as it comes closer. Kinetic stereopsis and increase in size work together, but in research must of course be studied separately.

FUSION: VISION BELOW THE THRESHOLD OF STEREOSCOPIC VISION

In the chapter on the evolution of vision we learned that stereoscopic vision is the *raison d'être* of binocular vision. When there is no visible depth, in principle 'oblique connections' do not function. Fusion then only consists of the merging of cortical elements which represent the same direction for both eyes, thus having no disparity.

RANGE OF FUSION

To direct both eyes with great precision onto the fixation point, the eyes are provided with a delicate motor system. The slightest disturbance of bifoveal fixation is corrected by movements of the two eyes in opposite directions. This is called *motor fusion*. The eyes can make vertical, horizontal and torsional movements. The amplitude of these movements is generally only a few degrees; the movement is slow, in the vertical direction even less than one degree per second.

Convergence is a disjunctive movement which falls into a special category, not only because of its large amplitude and, compared with other fusion movements, rapidity. It is the only disjunctive movement which can be carried out voluntarily. In addition, convergence forms part of the 'proximity synkinesis,' also called the 'near triad': convergence is associated with constriction of the pupil (miosis) and accommodation.

An obvious way to examine the fusion movements is to deregulate the binocular position of the eyes by putting prisms in front of them. The fact that the deregulation is temporary and the eyes adjust to the prisms within a few days does not invalidate the examination described below. For the sake of brevity, I restrict myself to base-out prisms (which force the eyes to converge) and base-in prisms (which cause divergence of the eyes). From the strength of the prisms which just fail to cause diplopia, the range of fusion can be measured.

THE FUSION CURVE AND THE MOTOR ROLE OF DISPARITY

The fusion movements caused by prisms usually fail to overcome the disparity completely. A little disparity remains, which increases as the forced fusion movements become greater. In these circumstances, therefore, we do not look with corresponding points, but with disparate points. There is maximum disparity at the point where the fusion is most strained, thus on the threshold of diplopia. We call this very slight disparity-induced increase of the total range of fusion the *range of sensory fusion*. The range of disparity is the same as that found in depth perception. Because the disparity by fusion is identical throughout the whole visual field, stereoscopic phenomena do not occur.

The residual disparity can be measured by a simple test when prisms of various strengths are put in front of the eyes (Fig. 7.18). In a small central field, in which there are no stimuli to horizontal fusion, two vernier lines are introduced which are movable in relation to each other; one can be seen by one eye and the other by the other (a method that was used for the determination of the horopter). When the subject is looking with disparate points instead of corresponding points, the vernier lines have to be placed obliquely one above the other in order to be seen as one line. The connection between the wrong position of the eyes forced by the prism and the residual disparity can be seen in the *fusion curve* (Fig. 7.19). On forced divergence the eyes remain not more than about twenty minutes of arc behind: *esodisparity*. On forced convergence *exodisparity* occurs. The sum of the maximum eso- and

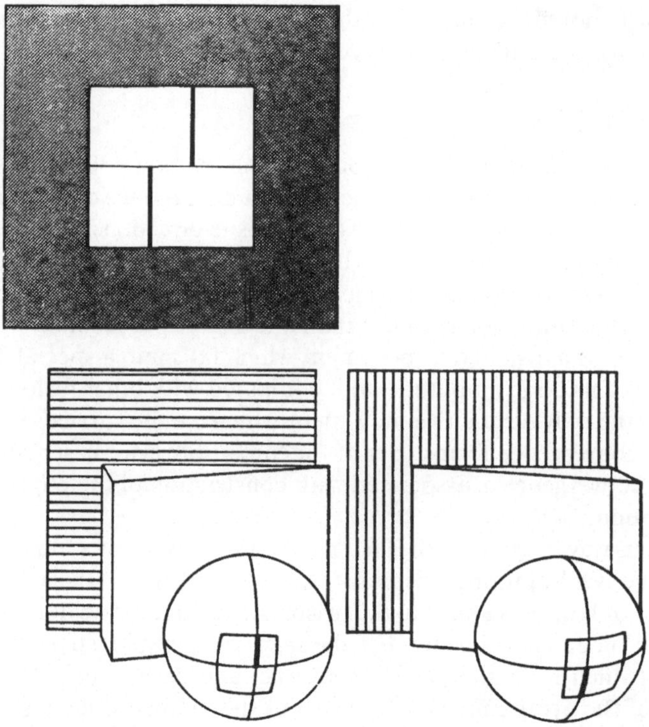

Fig. 7.18. Exodisparity in prismatically-induced convergence. The polarized vernier lines are haploscopically imaged on corresponding vertical meridians. The eyes are forced to converge by interposition of base-out prisms. The eyes lag slightly (exodisparity) and the fusion targets are fused, although they are imaged on non-corresponding points. Above: target with movable vernier lines. Below: eyes, prisms and polaroid plates.

exodisparities gives the range of the oblique connections in the given circumstances (see p. 94).

From diagram 7.2 we have learned that disparity, oblique connections, have a motor effect. Exodisparity causes convergence, and esodisparity causes divergence. It is tempting to assume that the exodisparity at the right side of the fusion curve gives motor support to convergence, and that, on the other hand, the esodisparity on the left side of the curve supports (or even generates) the movement of divergence.

But during a long trajectory of the forced convergence, the subject continues to look with corresponding points: the curve remains horizontal for a long time. That suggests that convergence has a special position among (or perhaps better, alongside) the fusion movements. In rare neurological conditions the convergence may become paralysed; in these cases the horizontal fusion curve is symmetrical and the fusion in the convergent direction behaves in the same way as the fusion in the divergent direction (dotted line in Fig. 7.19). Vertical fusion also has a curve like the dotted line in Figure 7.19. All these observations argue in favour of the hypothesis that fusion (except convergence) is controlled by disparity.

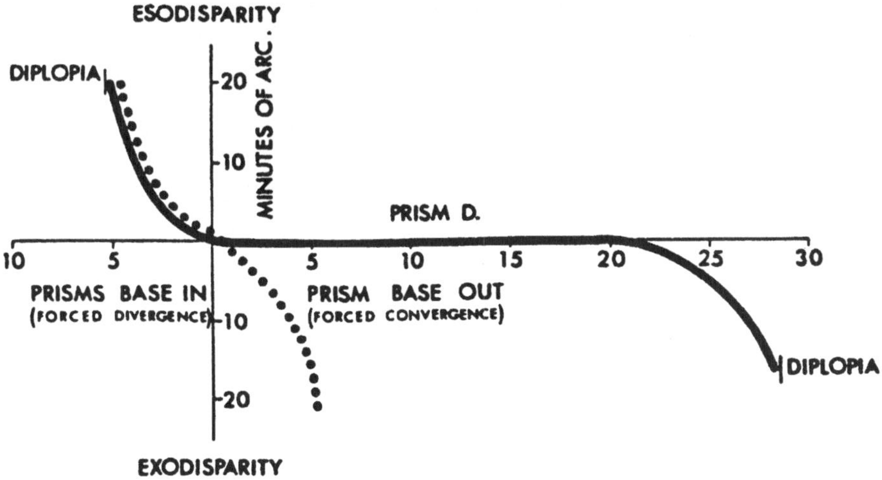

Fig. 7.19. The fusion curve. Horizontal fusion is possible between a divergent (base-in) prism of 4 PD (prism dioptre = approx. 1/2 degree) and a convergent (base-out) prism of 28 PD. The total fusional amplitude is 32 PD. In prismatically-induced divergence there is a maximum esodisparity of 20 minutes of arc; in prismatically-induced convergence the maximum exodisparity is also 20 minutes of arc. The distance between maximum eso- and exodisparity is thus 40 minutes of arc. In the given experimental setting this is the distance between the two diplopia thresholds.

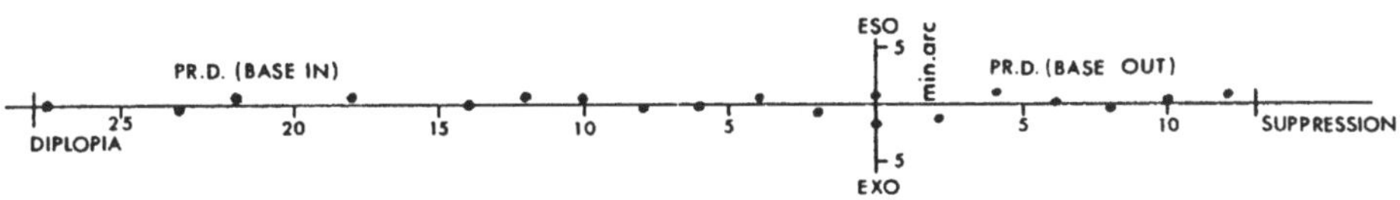

Fig. 7.20. Periodic divergent squint. Very weak binocular vision; no 'oblique links,' no stereoscopic vision.

In pathological cases oblique connections have failed to develop. Binocular vision is weak (with a tendency to look only with one eye) and there is no stereopsis. The fusion curve in such cases is completely flat (Fig. 7.20). Not disparity-controlled fusion, but only convergence keeps the eyes in the proper position.

RIVALRY, SUPPRESSION AND DOMINANCE

When the contours of the images received by the two eye are dissimilar and cannot be combined by stereoscopy or fusion, rivalry ensues. The two patterns fight for the supremacy in perception (Fig. 7.21). The contours which lose the battle are 'suppressed.' Suppression is an obstacle to binocular vision but is, as will be argued in a later section, at the same time a necessary condition for stereopsis.

When contours are absent, images in the right and left eyes which only differ in brightness or colour can be combined. When the colours are different binocular

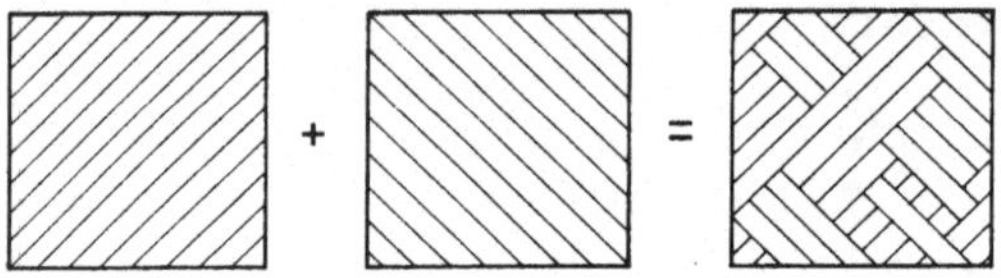

Fig. 7.21. Rivalry. On stimulation of corresponding points with equivalent but not identical contours. When the contours are not equivalent one of the images is completely suppressed.

Fig. 7.22. A simple stereogram ('Panum's limiting case'). The left line is seen in two directions. Nothing changes in the depth sensation if the separate line (with a dot) is combined with the right (front) or the left (back) line.

colour mixing occurs. When there are local differences in brightness 'binocular gloss' arises; the combination of the two images gives a metallic sheen.

DOMINANCE

Naturally, when the image in one eye is completely dominant over the other, stereopsis is impossible. We have then entered the realm of pathology. In healthy eyes dominance is rare. Microscopists used to look through microscopes with one eye-piece. Many of them learned to keep the eye open which was not looking through the eye-piece. But in normal circumstances there is a subtle equilibrium. That signifies that the binocular localisation is strictly intermediate. This is not altered by the fact that most people have a 'master eye,' which dominates when the choice between the eyes is *forced*. When one points at an object seen with two eyes and then closes the two eyes successively, the object, finger and master eye are found to be in one line. This form of dominance plays no part in binocular vision.

THE PSYCHOPHYSICS OF STEREOGRAMS

As Wheatstone demonstrated, two spatial points can be seen as one in spite of the fact that the two eyes individually see them in different directions. The opposite is also true: one spatial point can be localised in two different directions, although in each eye only one retinal point is stimulated. That can be concluded from the stereogram in Figure 7.22. Another important fact can also be learnt from the stereogram: that nothing changes in the depth sensation if the separate line (with a dot),

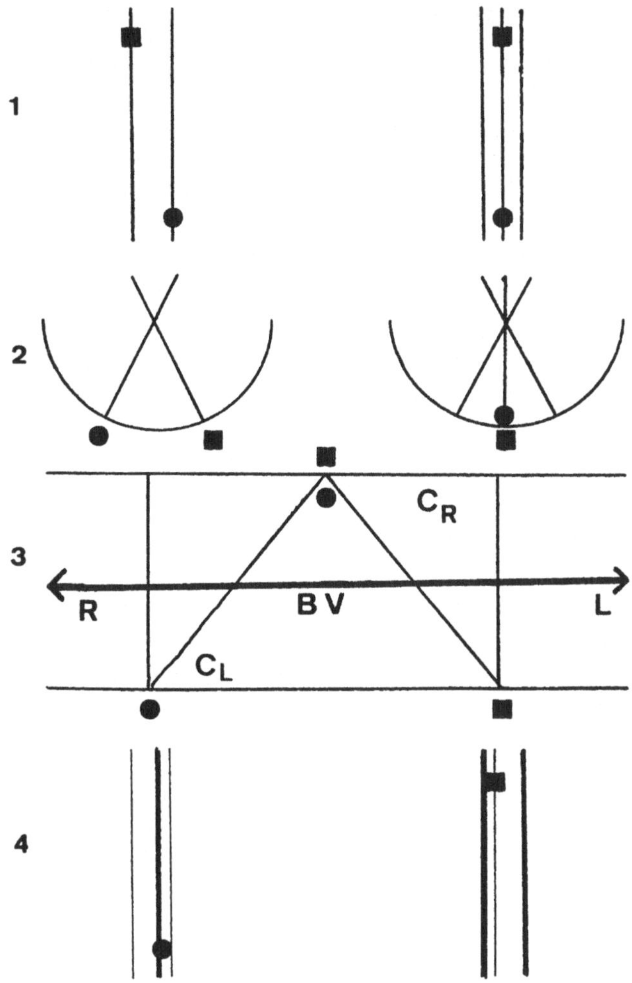

Fig. 7.23. 'Displacement.' From above to below: (1) stereogram; (2) retinal image; (3) on the line BV the circle is localized to the right, the cube to the left; (4) subjective appearance.

through variation in the degree of convergence, is combined binocularly with the front or the back line: convergence and disparity are equivalent, as already stated.

The stereogram in Figure 7.23 is also worth studying. When one tries to combine the middle line in the right image with the right line in the left image (by fusion of the circles), one sees the middle line displaced to the front and to the right. On an attempt to combine the middle line of the right image with the left line of the left image (by fusion of the squares), one sees the middle line displaced backwards and to the left. The displacement of the middle line has the impressive name of 'allelotropia,' which means nothing more than that the binocular localisation is intermediate. The diagram makes this clear.

JULESZ' RANDOM DOTS PATTERN

When stereophotography was popular—and for a long time afterwards—stereoscopy was considered to be a higher psychical process. Stereoscopy was produced by an unconscious comparison of the two perspectives from which the outside world was seen. In Duke-Elder's *System of Ophthalmology* (1958–1976), the influential text-book of the fifties, this is strikingly expressed: 'It is as though each image were seen by one of two observers with similar vision, and as though the minds of the two observers were combined into a single mind.'

The elementary structure in Figure 7.22 makes one doubt the necessity of explaining depth perception as the combination of 'two souls in one breast.' Intelligent minds had presumed for a long time that a physiological approach to depth perception was possible. The discovery of the 'disparity detectors' by Barlow et al. (1967) first definitely drew attention to the existence of elementary construction units for depth perception (p. 110).

Bela Julesz (1964) demonstrated elegantly that monocular recognition of a *pattern* is not necessary for depth perception. He made stereograms (Fig. 7.24) with a computer which he called Random Dot Patterns. Figure 7.25 shows how these stereograms were made. In the centre of one of the plates the A-B motive is shifted to the right. The available space is then filled with X-Y. On binocular fusion one sees a central square in depth (Fig. 7.26). Thus depth perception arises without recognition of the two different plates, because neither of the plates reveals in any way what will appear after the combination of the images.

Julesz, with his RDPs, gave a new impulse to the psychological study of depth perception. Much of his work, and that of his associates, is assembled in the book *Principles of Cyclopean Perception* (1971). The hero of the title is the wicked giant Polyphemus, a Cyclops with one eye in the middle of his forehead. Odysseus and his companions only just managed to escape from him. The Cyclops is an attractive metaphor for (binocular) single vision. The 'cyclopean eye' was already popular

Fig. 7.24. Random Dot Stereogram according to Julesz (1964). The square that can be seen stereoscopically, is not visible in the separate plates.

with scolars in the nineteenth century, as a virtual eye between the two real eyes. For Julesz, 'cyclopean vision' is nothing more than a metaphor for seeing RDPs.

It is worth while to study Julesz' RDPs more closely. The fusion of the two images by the combination of the peripheral contours and details is no problem. When one has found the right degree of convergence—mainly by fixating on the outlines of

1	0	1	0	1	0	0	1	0	1
1	0	0	1	0	1	0	1	0	0
0	0	1	1	0	1	1	0	1	0
0	1	0	Y	A	A	B	B	0	1
1	1	1	X	B	A	B	A	0	1
0	0	1	X	A	A	B	A	1	0
1	1	1	Y	B	B	A	B	0	1
1	0	0	1	1	0	1	1	0	1
1	1	0	0	1	1	0	1	1	1
0	1	0	0	0	1	1	1	1	0

1	0	1	0	1	0	0	1	0	1
1	0	0	1	0	1	0	1	0	0
0	0	1	1	0	1	1	0	1	0
0	1	0	A	A	B	B	0	0	1
1	1	1	B	A	B	A	0	0	1
0	0	1	A	A	B	A	0	1	0
1	1	1	B	B	A	B	0	0	1
1	0	0	1	1	0	1	1	0	1
1	1	0	0	1	1	0	1	1	1
0	1	0	0	0	1	1	1	1	0

Fig. 7.25. Construction of a random-dot stereogram. The central A-B square in the right plate has been shifted to the right in the left plate.

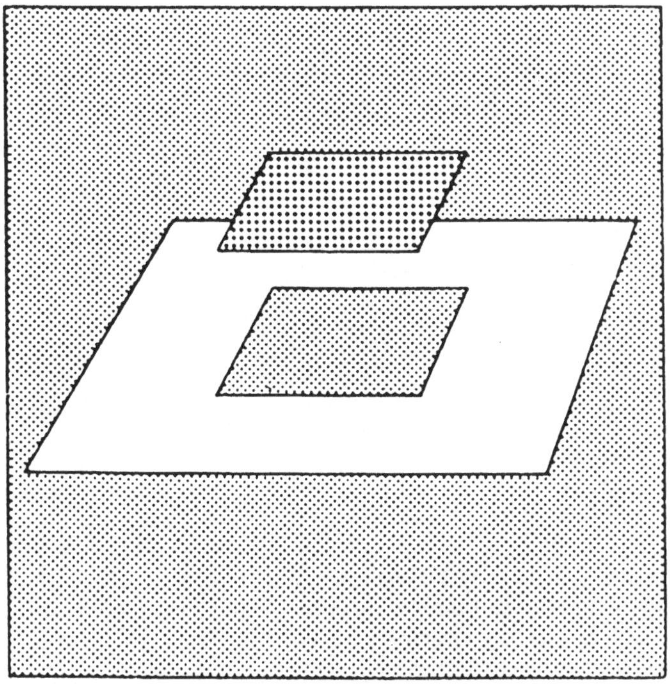

Fig. 7.26. Stereo-effect of Figure 7.14 on underconvergence.

the two figures—one can easily see the peripheries in one plane. But how does the visual system find the right connection between all those tiny central figures, in such a way that a central square is seen in depth? The first step is undoubtedly the refusal of the combination of dissimilar elements of the image. Elements of an image can be dissimilar in two ways: by differences in brightness (black and white) or by differences in shape (e.g., single or double blocks). Binocular vision can use the mechanism of rivalry for this purpose. But not much is achieved in this way. Because which single black block corresponds with which single black block in the other plate? The number of possible combinations of black blocks is immense. Figure 7.27 gives an impression of this. Two halves of an RDP are laid on top of each

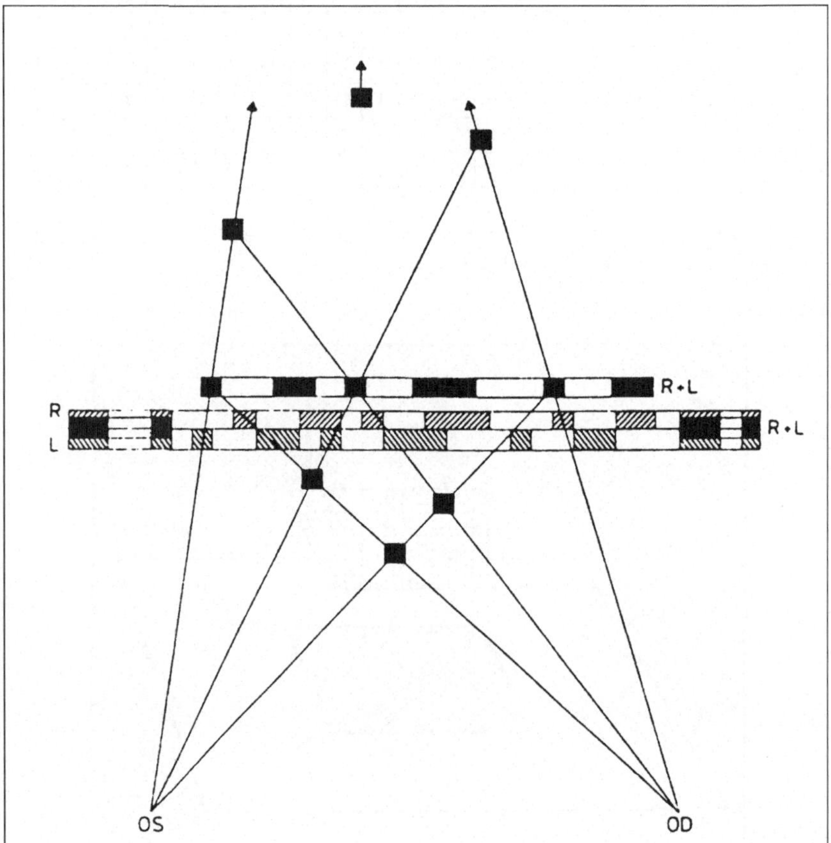

Fig. 7.27. Rivalry and globality. Two superimposed random dot stereograms. The stereograms presented to the right and left eyes are shaded by thin lines (R, L) and the stereoscopic image (R + L) is black. The upper stereogram is seen by the right eye, the lower by the left eye. The central field lies two blocks farther to the right in the upper pattern. *Rivalry*: single white and black blocks are not fused. *Globality*: fusion of single black blocks could result in depth perception at various distances. But blocks are seen only in one plane behind the frame.

other. Peripherally the plates are identical. The contours stimulate corresponding points (R + L). At the centre the figures in the right stereogram are shifted two blocks to the right relative to the figures on the left. When the left eye looks at three square black blocks in the left stereogram, and the right eye at three in the right stereogram, no less than nine blocks are projected in space. Then follows the next step: it is seen that three of these nine blocks lie in the same plane. These three are chosen for the binocular image (R + L). They join hands, as it were, and together drive the six 'ghost images' away. Julesz calls this process 'globalisation,' the union of local depth data into one. From the simple example in Figure 7.27 it can be clearly seen how incredibly complicated the process must be by which, in Figure 7.24 with so many blocks, a central square can be recognized. An important part in this process is played by the *horror profundi*, the binocular system's dislike of depth, associated with facilitation of binocular elements of the image which lie in one plane.

That even becomes clear in the case of two elements of the image, in Krol and Van de Grind's 'two-nail illusion' (Fig. 7.28). Two identical nails, one behind the other, are seen as two nails *next to each other*. The explanation of the illusion is shown in Figure 7.29. The horror profundi is an effective form of repulsion: the majority of points in space usually lie at the same depth; they form part of a plane that is wholly seen at a certain depth.

At first, the ingenious Julesz patterns make a rather artificial impression. But the contrary is true. Someone who looks with one eye at the leaves above his head in a wood, sees a great number of leaves without depth. With both eyes open he discovers that the leaves are arranged in layers, depending on the branches to which they are attached. Another example: someone who makes an ordinary aerial photograph of a flat terrain with tanks which are covered by camouflage nets, sees nothing special. But on a stereo-photograph the depth differences in the camouflage nets are immediately recognized.

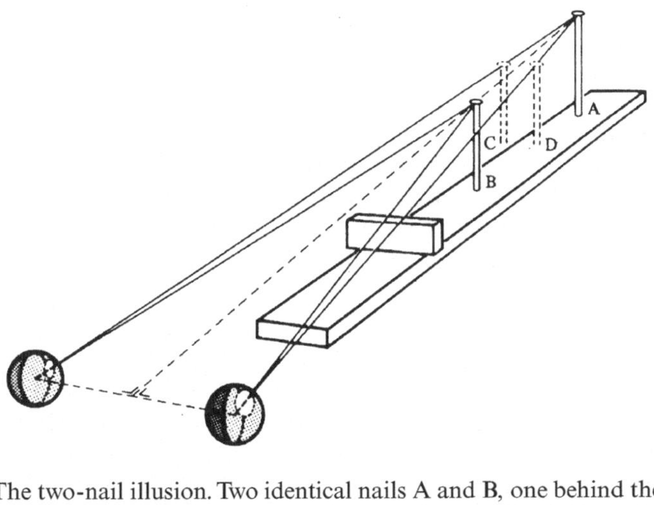

Fig. 7.28. The two-nail illusion. Two identical nails A and B, one behind the other in the median plane, are seen as two nails C and D next to each other (Krol & Van de Grint, 1980).

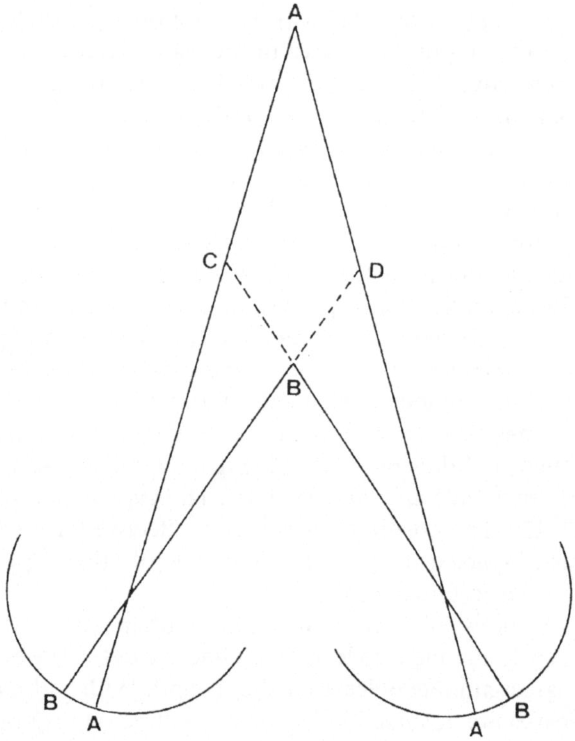

Fig. 7.29. Explanation of the two-nail illusion. Nails C and D both arise by fusion of nails A and B. The images C and D have no retinal disparity and are therefore seen in one frontal plane (between A and B).

STEREOSCOPY AND VERGENCE

From Wheatstone to Julesz it has been mainly psychological investigation that has given us insight into stereoscopy. Disparity was the main point of interest. Less attention was given to depth perception as a sensorimotor process. Investigation of vergence as the motor effect of disparity is indeed difficult. In the first place, vergence movements have a relatively small amplitude; secondly, there is the discouraging discovery that there is a discrepancy between the empirical horopter and the vergence; and finally, there is the fact that perception of depth can occur in situations in which even diplopia exists. All this indicates that disparity and vergence are not very well attuned.

But it is important to remember that there are two types of stereopsis: sensitive static stereopsis and the much less precise kinetic stereopsis. Depth perception and vergence will be better co-ordinated during an eye operation than during a boxing match. It is certain that vergence in static stereopsis has a high degree of precision. Determination of the fusion curve by the vernier method (Fig. 7.19) has shown that vergence is very stable and can be easily measured subjectively with an accuracy of one minute of arc.

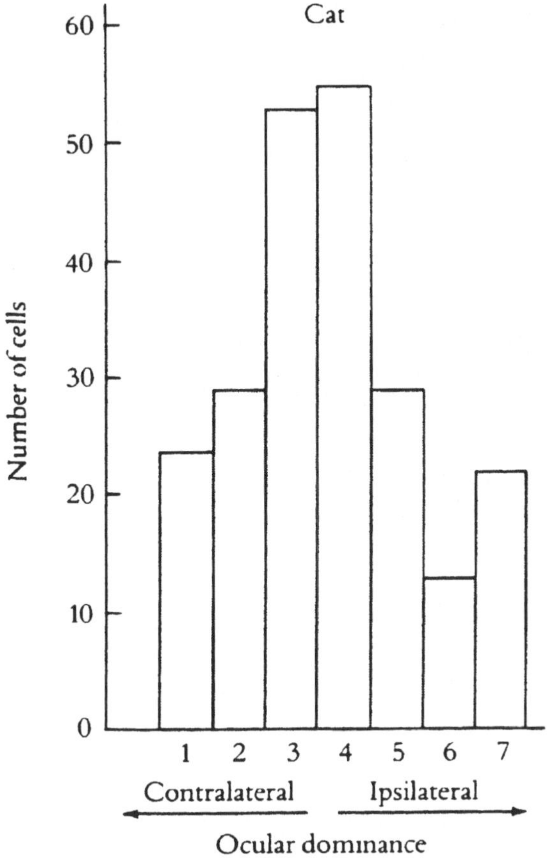

Fig. 7.30. Ocular dominance. The cells in column 1 can only be stimulated by impulses from the contralateral eye, the cells in column 7 only from the ipsilateral eye. The cells in column 4 are equally sensitive to impulses from both eyes (Hubel, 1988).

THE NEUROPHYSIOLOGY OF BINOCULAR VISION

In the section on visual acuity, the technique of the neurophysiological investigation of the visual system was explained. It was found possible to chart the receptive fields of individual cells in the visual cortex. An important finding was reported: the cells are sensitive to linear stimuli with a certain orientation in the visual field. Another, no less important, discovery by Hubel and Wiesel has not yet been mentioned: a great many cells, even the large majority, can be activated by stimuli from both the right and the left eye. Some cells give an equal reaction to stimulation from either eye, others react more strongly to stimuli from one eye than the other, others again can only be stimulated monocularly (Fig. 7.30). Still more interesting is the fact that cells also exist which are insensitive to monocular stimuli but give a strong response to binocular stimulation. It is easy to assume that it is these cells that are the neurophysiological correlate of binocular stereoscopic vision. In the chapter on visual

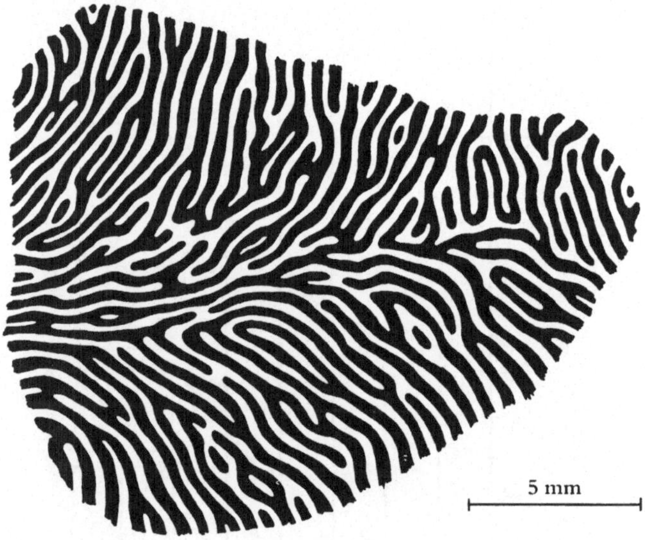

Fig. 7.31. Dominance columns in the visual cortex. Obtained by autoradiography after injection of a radio-active preparation into one eye. Reconstruction by Le Vay (Hubel, 1988).

acuity we saw that cells with the same orientation were to be found in one column in the visual cortex. On the other hand, if the electrode is thrust into the cortex in the direction parallel to the surface, cells are found with different orientations. But more than that is found: it is possible that first cells are encountered which are more strongly activated by one eye and then cells for which the other eye is dominant (Fig. 7.31). In the visual cortex there are *dominance columns* arranged side by side in bands. The columns in the visual cortex do not only have one orientation, but also have predominantly monocular dominance. Figure 7.31, in which dominance bands can be seen, was produced as follows: a month before anatomical examination of the brain of an ape, a radio-active substance was injected into one of its eyes. The substance diffused along the visual pathways to the visual cortex. A photograph of a flat slice of the visual cortex produced the dominance pattern shown.

In 1967 Barlow and his associates made an important discovery. They were examining the receptive fields of cells in the visual cortex of the cat. It appeared that binocular cells were attuned to various disparities. Bishop's (idealised) diagram (Fig. 7.32) illustrates the principle. Suppose that an anaesthetised cat converges its eyes to the fixation point shown on the diagram. The curved plane through that point is then the cat's horopter. If a binocular cell has 'normal correspondence,' the receptive fields of that cell coincide with the horopter. That is the case for cell 2 in diagram A. On the other hand, the receptive fields of cell 3 (diagram B) coincide in front of the horopter and those of cell 1 (diagram C) behind it. Neither of these cells can be activated by a stimulus on the horopter.

Some depth cells are attuned to a large degree of disparity, others to a small degree. It is clear that the disparity detectors form the neurophysiological substratum of stereoscopic depth perception and of the 'oblique connections' in my diagram.

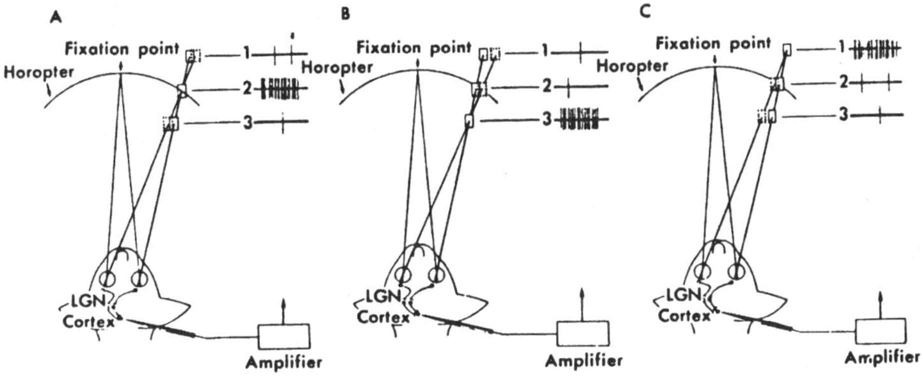

Fig. 7.32. Scheme showing how binocular information can be coded by neurons in cat visual cortex. (A) Maximal firing of binocularly activated neuron occurs when the two monocular receptive fields are in register and can be stimulated simultaneously, tracing 2. Being in register on the horopter, this receptive field pair has zero disparity, that is, they are corresponding. (B) Receptive field pair having convergent disparity; maximal firing, tracing 3. (C) Receptive field pair having divergent disparity; maximal firing, tracing 1 (from Bishop, 1975).

There appears to be a certain amount of agreement between the sensitivity to disparity of the depth cells and the sensitivity, as measured by animal psychology, of (static) stereoscopic vision.

Later it became apparent that the rougher kinetic depth perception follows a separate path in the nervous system. Some think that this even starts in the retina. According to them, static stereoscopy originates in the beta-cells in the retina and the slow, precise parvocellular system in the LGN, while kinetic depth perception is brought about via the rapid but inexact alpha-cellular and magnocellular system. The disparity detectors of kinetic depth perception are also different. They are, in a wide range of disparity, only sensitive to either crossed or uncrossed disparity. Poggio et al. (1988) performed experiments on alert, trained macaque monkeys and inventoried six types of binocular neurons (Fig. 7.33): neurons that are stimulated by nondisparity (TO) or inhibited by nondisparity (TI), that have precisely attuned sensitivity to near (TN) or distant (TF), and neurons with roughly attuned sensitivity to near (NE) or distant (FA).

It is tempting to give each of these six types of neurons a specific function in binocular vision: the TO neurons as the basis of fusion, the TI neurons as the substratum of rivalry, the TN and TF neurons as the performers of static stereopsis and the NE and FA neurons as the substratum of inexact kinetic stersopsis.

THE NEUROPHYSIOLOGY OF DISJUNCTIVE MOVEMENTS

Poggio's figures show us how far neurophysiological analysis has advanced in the field of the differentiation and central processing of afferent stimuli. But the neurophysiology of disjunctive movements, on the other hand, is a neglected area. Of course it is clear to everyone that signals from the disparity detectors lead

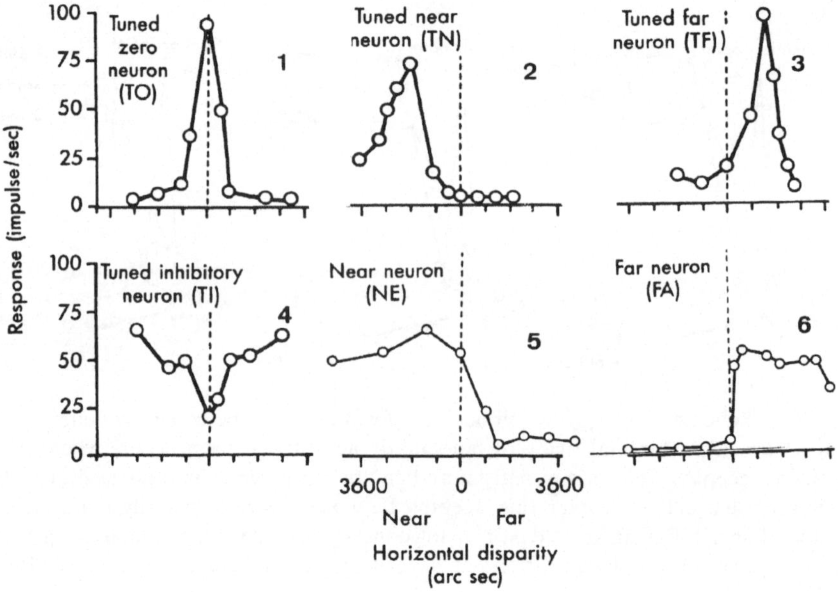

Fig. 7.33. Disparity detectors in area V1 of alert macaques trained to maintain fixation on a near target. (1) sharply tuned zero-disparity neurons; (2 and 3) sharply tuned 'far' and 'near' detectors; (4) inhibitory neurons; (5 and 6) 'near' and 'far' neurons with much flatter tuning (After Poggio et al., 1988).

to disjunctive movements, and it is probable that these signals are bundled into motor impulses in higher visual areas. The areas V3 and V3a in the ape have four times as many 'stereoneurons' as 'flat binocular neurons.' But the paths along which the disjunctive impulses reach the eye muscles are unknown. Although it should be reported that Jampel, as early as 1959, found a parieto-occipital area in apes which on stimulation produced convergence, accommodation and constriction of the pupil. Pathology has taught us that convergence may be exclusively paralysed by lesions in the midbrain. This is in agreement with Figures 7.1 and 7.2, in which different centres are assumed for conjugate and disjunctive eye movements. Still less is known about vertical and torsional fusion movements. The combination of vertical fusion movements with torsion and nystagmus suggests a relationship with primitive labyrinthine reflexes.

8. The Pathology of Binocular Depth Perception: Squint and Amblyopia

SQUINT (STRABISMUS)

Nature has accepted many sacrifices in the interests of stereoscopic vision. Two laterally placed eyes without—or almost without—a binocular field of vision give a panoramic view without depth perception. Two frontally placed eyes have a smaller visual field but can see depth. Some animals, such as herbivores, have chosen the wide view; others, like apes, who must be able to precisely estimate the distance to the next branch, have chosen depth perception. Man has also been provided with eyes like that. He learned to walk upright and to use his hands with self-made instruments for numerous purposes. Stereoscopic vision, so extremely accurate at the distance of the hands, was of great importance. Absence of stereopsis must have been a dangerous failing for a primitive human being.

For the man of today the loss of binocular vision, usually associated with squint, is not so important any more. His greatest risk is a traffic accident, which cannot be prevented by stereoscopy. His greatest passion is the television, with a flat picture without depth effects. His chief occupation is filling in forms, but paper is flat and undemanding. You probably will not find good dentists among people with a squint, or good ophthalmic surgeons. But generally speaking it is the disfiguring position of the eyes, not the loss of depth perception, which drives the squinter to the doctor.

A SHORT HISTORY OF SQUINT[1]

In folklore, the squinting eye is traditionally the 'evil eye' (*oculus fascinus*). In primitive societies the evil eye is an important cause of sickness and death. Someone who looks squint-eyed looks with hatred at someone who is better off, a farmer with more land, a woman of great beauty. It is all the more remarkable that among the Mayas of Central-America a squint was considered a sign of beauty. Was that because a squint was common and people were proud of it as a racial characteristic? The Mayas even tried to create a squint by hanging a ball between the eyes of small children (Fig. 8.1). Perhaps this method was successful: when the first Spanish

[1] Crone, 1964.

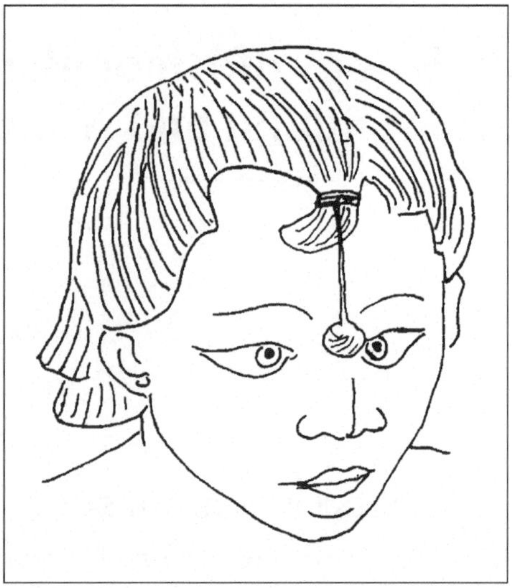

Fig. 8.1. Induced squint in Mayas.

scouts penetrated into Yucatan two Mayas were taken prisoner. And both of them, according to the chronicle writer Bernal Diaz de Castillo, had a squint!

Paulus of Aegina (623–690), a doctor in Alexandria, was the first to think of a rational treatment of squint: a mask with eyeholes positioned in such a way that the squinting eye was forced to correct its position. This treatment didn't help, but a thousand years later no advance had been made, if one looks at Figure 8.2 taken from Georg Bartisch (1583), the man who wrote the first European textbook of ophthalmology. In 1585 Jacques Guillemeau published the second textbook. His advice was to put drops of turtle or pigeon blood into the squinting eye. Bannister, one of Guillemeau's followers, wrote about squint in 1622: 'I have seen it proceed in some, of having too much company with woman, the excess whereof doeth marvelously scatter the spirits. But commonly it is a maladie most incident into children presently after their birth, through the negligence of the Nurce, who setteth the cradle, in which the infant lieth, on the side of the light.'

The naturalist George-Louis Leclerc, comte de Buffon (1707–1788), the author of the *Histoire naturelle générale et particulière* in 44 volumes, came closer to the truth. He squinted himself and blamed that on poor vision in one eye. The incorrect position of the eyes was due to an attempt to be as little troubled as possible by the weak eye; the weak eye was forced to flee!

A new idea, that squint could be cured by an operation, came from the famous Chevalier John Taylor (1703–1772), the knight errant of ophthalmology. His shrewdness was mentioned in the context of the optic chiasma (p. 90), now we must pay some attention to his knavery. Taylor travelled with his retinue through the courts and cities of Europe in a coach which was decorated with painted eyes. It is probable that he understood the art of healing less well than the art of advertising. He extracted the last pennies from the pockets of many blind victims. Frederick the

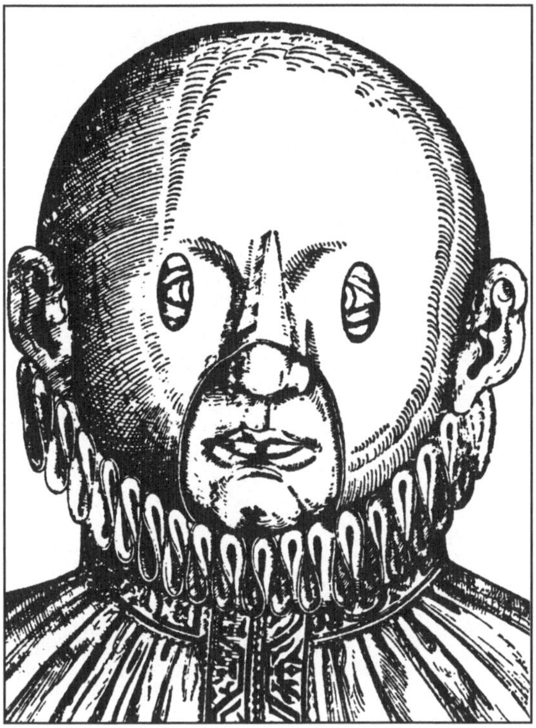

Fig. 8.2. Treatment of squint by Georg Bartisch (1583).

Great threatened to hang him if he dared to touch any of his subjects. Taylor maltreated Bach's eyes so drastically that he died in misery shortly afterwards, but not before he had finished dictating his last work 'Vor deinen Thron tret ich hiemit.' Händel's experience was not very different, he was also operated on by Taylor. An article appeared in the paper 'On the recovery of Sight of the Celebrated Mr Handel, by the Chevalier Taylor.' But Händel also became blind and died within a few months.

As far as the squint operation is concerned: Taylor only made a snip in the conjunctiva of one eye, ostensibly to cut a nerve going to an eye muscle. He bandaged that eye, so that the other eye took up a straight position, and left the bandage on until he had ridden away in his coach. When Taylor played this trick in Rouen, the anatomist Lecat decided to teach him a lesson. Taylor invited Lecat to a banquet and told him about his squint operation. Lecat then let a covered dish be carried in which Taylor had not ordered: it was a cleft human head in which the nerves of the eye muscles had been dissected out. The knight made a poor showing, because none of the nerves lay directly under the conjunctiva.

It was not until a hundred years later that Dieffenbach did the first operation on an eye muscle (1839). In cases of convergent squint he cut the tendon of the medial rectus muscle (Fig. 8.3). Often the eye turned too far in the opposite direction and the squint was uglier than before. Dieffenbach's victims were known as

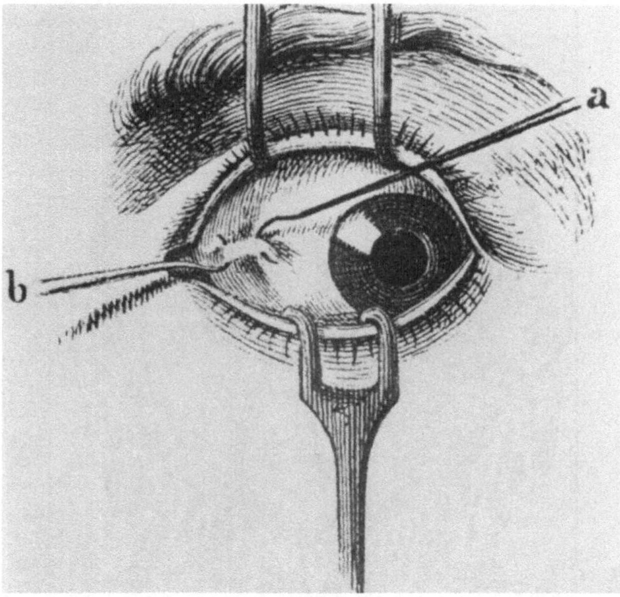

Fig. 8.3. Dieffenbach's tenotomy (1839). The tendon of the eye muscle is held by a hook and only needs to be cut.

'Dieffenbachers' in Berlin. (Later a technically improved operation became the most important treatment of squint.)

This was the right moment to consider squint more deeply. It was Cornelis Franciscus Donders who made the connection between convergent squint and long-sightedness (1864). His train of thought was simple: when a hypermetropic child (a child with eyes which have insufficient refractive power and who thus needs positive glasses to see properly) wants to see well, it has to accommodate, even when it is looking into the distance. The convergence associated by nature with accommodation forces the eyes into the convergent position. The child therefore has to choose between clear vision with one eye or hazy vision with two eyes. Donders was able to cure many children with glasses, but far from all of them. (Glasses are still often prescribed to overcome or decrease the squint.)

Émile Javal (1839–1907) approached squint in a different way. Starting from the work of his fellow-countryman Buffon, he laid emphasis on the inequality of the eyes and disturbances of binocular vision. He began his career as mining engineer, but when his squinting sister was threatened with an operation he decided to study medicine and to treat her with a stereoscope (Fig. 8.4). The stereoscope, which had only recently become popular, had fascinated Javal as a child. It seemed to him to be the most suitable instrument to get the straying binocular vision back onto the rails. Javal sometimes practised in daily sessions with a child for months on end. The child was taken away from school and placed in the care of a governess who also had to spend several hours a day practising. Later, Javal summarized his work in his famous *Manuel du strabisme* (1896). He had to admit that he had only

§ 54. **Stéréoscope à charnière.** — Malgré la précaution que nous avons prise d'augmenter le champ du stéréoscope par l'emploi de lentilles à foyers relativement courts, il arrive souvent que la déviation est trop forte pour qu'on puisse faire usage du stéréoscope à lentilles. C'est alors qu'on trouve avantage à employer mon stéréoscope à charnière.

Cet instrument, sous sa forme la plus récente, a été calculé pour amener les images à environ 16 centimètres des yeux, nécessitant ainsi une accommodation d'environ six dioptrics. Cette dimension a été choisie pour rendre les déviations du regard obtenues dans cet instrument facilement comparables à celles dans un stéréoscope ordinaire, muni de verres de six pouces.

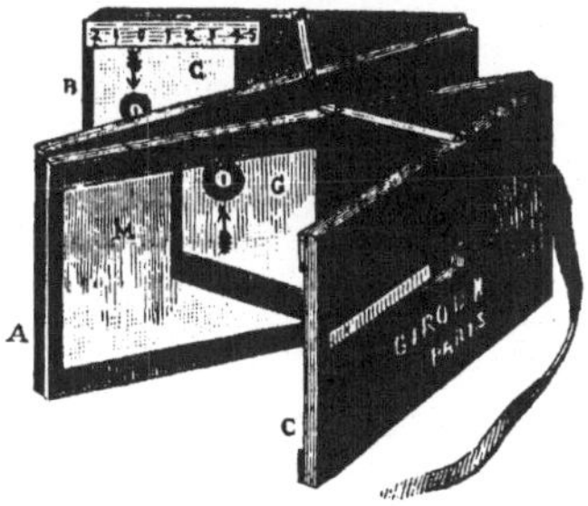

Fig. 36.

Fig. 8.4. Javal's hinged stereoscope (1896). The angle between the mirrors, which was 90° by Wheatstone, can be adjusted to the incorrect position of the eyes.

succeeded in a limited number of cases in restoring the binocular vision. The greatest obstacle was the 'anomalous binocular vision.'

ABNORMAL BINOCULAR VISION

There are various sorts of squint, but in most cases the eyes deviate in the convergent direction. In the following section I shall restrict myself to convergent squint. The angle of squint (the wrong position of the eyes) can be small (a fraction of a degree) but also very large, e.g., 40 degrees. A striking feature is that squinting children don't see double. That is due to suppression (where the angle of squint is large). When the angle is smaller, adaptation of binocular vision can make suppression partially unnecessary. When the angle is extremely small there is no suppression.

Compare the fusion curve of normal binocular vision (Fig. 7.19) with Figure 8.5. The angle of squint is extremely small, only 1/4 degree and is scarcely influenced by prisms. The diplopia-free zone (the range of sensory fusion) is rather small, so that a certain tendency to double vision and slightly reduced stereoscopic vision may be expected. But there is no suppression and there is adequate motor fusion. Binocular vision is achieved via 'oblique connections' and is therefore '*abnormal binocular vision*.' When binocular vision comes about through oblique, disparate, links, an impulse to divergence is to be expected (Fig. 7.2). That is indeed the case: When binocular vision is interrupted by putting a hand before one eye, that eye is seen to converge ('heterophoria').

When the angle of squint is larger, anomalous binocular vision becomes weaker. In view of the 'cortical enlargement,' the oblique connections in the centre of the visual field are more difficult to make. Foveal suppression arises in the squinting eye. The existence of anomalous binocular vision with an angle of squint of 7 degrees, for instance, can be demonstrated with Bagolini's striped glasses

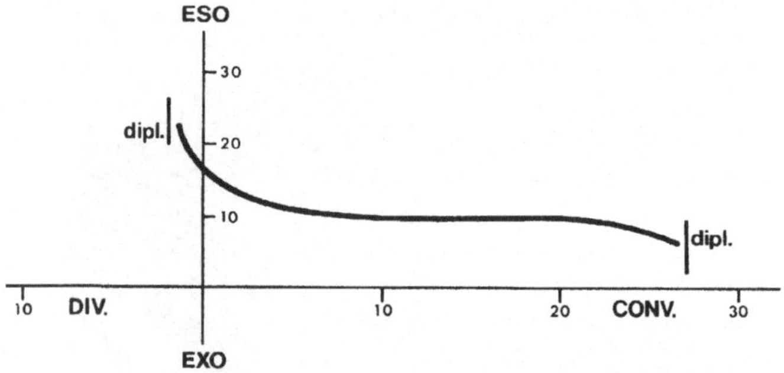

Fig. 8.5. Fusion curve of a patient with a convergent squint of 16 minutes of arc (on the vertical scale). The horizontal scale is in prism dioptres (1 PD = ±1/2 degree).

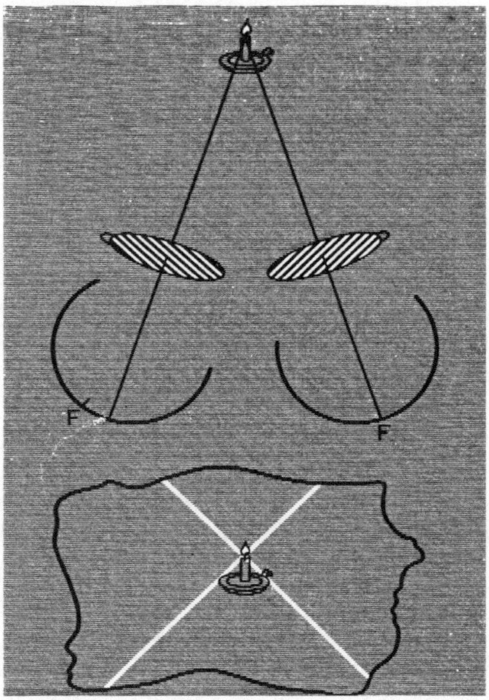

Fig. 8.6. Abnormal correspondence, demonstrated with Bagolini's striped glasses. Although the left eye is convergent, both stripes pass through the fixation point of the fixating eye.

(Fig. 8.6). Glasses with parallel, scarcely visible scratches turn a spot of light into a stripe. If a glass like this is placed in front of each eye, with the scratches in front of one eye perpendicular to the scratches in front of the other, both stripes are seen, in spite of the squint, to run through the fixation point of the fixating eye. This is called *'abnormal correspondence.'* It is the proof that the squinting eye still contributes to binocular vision. When the angle of squint is greater, this is no longer the case; suppression is then complete.

The attentive reader will be surprised that monocular stimuli (the vernier lines) are localised in the first case (with angle of 1/4 degree) according to the real position of the eye, while in the second case (with angle of 7 degrees) the stripe in Bagolini's test is localised wrongly by the squinting eye. The explanation is simple: in the first case each retina contributes equally to the (intermediate) binocular localisation. In the second case, the localisation of the straight eye is dominant; the squinting eye attunes its localisation to that of the fixating eye (Fig. 8.7).

THE CAUSE OF SQUINT

The cause of squint is unknown, although hypermetropia plays a role in a limited number of cases. Most authors leave this question open. In 1956 I assumed that there is a disturbance in the afferent part of the optic pathway (Crone & Velzeboer, 1956). This hypothesis seemed to be supported in the seventies, when squinting Siamese (albino) cats were found to have a defect in the uncrossed part of the optic tract. This neurological abnormality was also found in human albinos (who have abnormal binocular vision also).

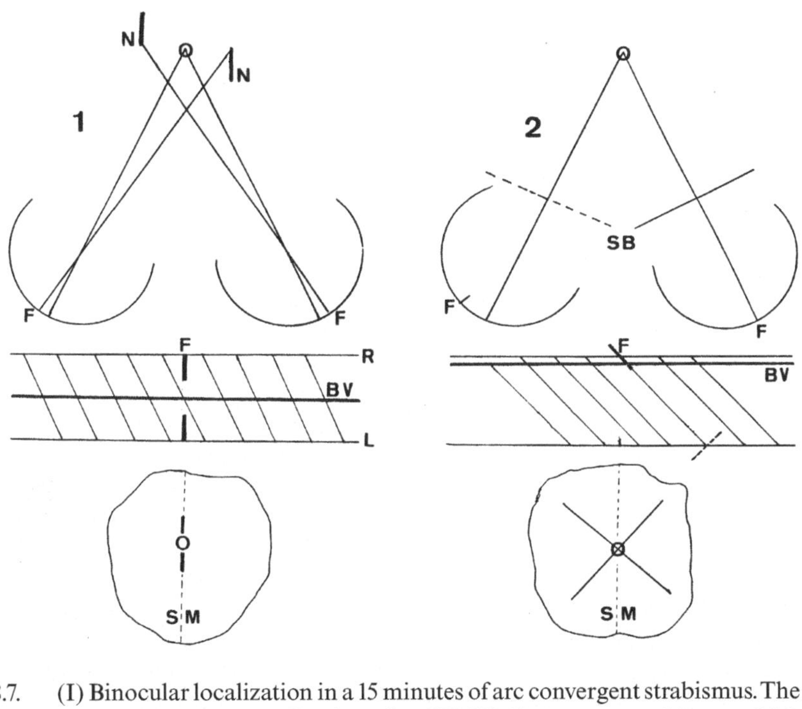

Fig. 8.7. (I) Binocular localization in a 15 minutes of arc convergent strabismus. The foveal nonius lines are localized intermediately on line BV. (II) Convergent strabismus of 5 degrees. The right eye fixates and dominates the localization (BV coincides with C_R). The left eye adapts its localization to the right eye.

With the limited examination methods then available, no abnormalities of the optic pathways were found in cases of ordinary squint without albinism. But an afferent disturbance is still possible. Recently a few patients have been described with squint and the absence of the chiasma, in which cases it is the crossed tracts that are missing[2].

Because no good animal model for squint exists, little is known about its neurophysiology. Animals have been made to squint artificially, and the development of abnormal binocular vision has been followed. In cats with induced vertical squint, binocular cells have been found which could be stimulated by a receptive field of one eye and also by a, vertically displaced, receptive field of the other eye.

THE ONTOGENY OF BINOCULAR VISION

As shown in Figure 8.8, a child is born with normal binocular correspondence. It has no choice, because the optic fibres from the LGN only project onto one cortical cell. Thus there are no 'oblique connections' and there is no stereoscopic vision. Studies have shown that stereoscopic vision appears rather suddenly around the

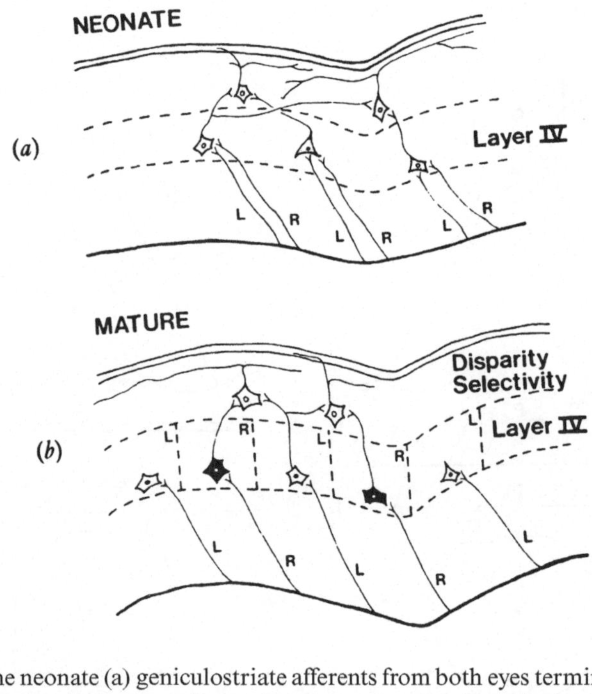

Fig. 8.8. In the neonate (a) geniculostriate afferents from both eyes terminate on the same cells in layer IV, thereby losing information about the eye of origin. In the mature brain (b) geniculostriate afferents are segregated on the basis of eye origin. Synapses between R and L cells may be disparity-selective (after Held, 1991).

---

[2] Apkarian et al., 1995.

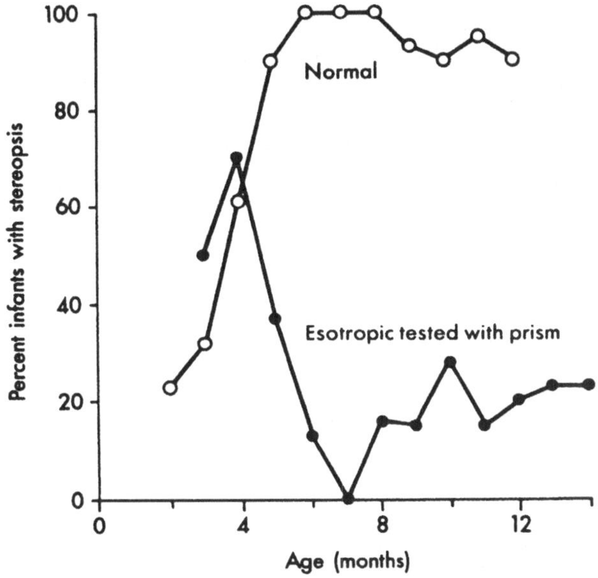

Fig. 8.9. Normal development of stereoscopic vision (open circles). Vulnerability of stereoscopic vision in squint (black circles) (after Birch & Stager, 1985).

fourth month. Figure 8.9 shows how stereoscopic vision is completed at about six months with the development of disparity detectors. In early squint stereoscopic vision is extremely vulnerable. If the angle of squint is corrected with prisms, it is at first possible to evoke stereoscopic vision, but after the age of five months this is no longer possible.

AMBLYOPIA

Amblyopia is the Greek word for 'dullsightedness'. The word was used formerly for many known and unknown forms of poor sight, but has now a well-defined meaning. It is a disturbance of vision which appears when the eye misses visual experience in the first years of life. The reduction in the visual acuity can be slight, but also so extreme that the eye is useless. The usual cause is unilateral squint. Buffon already knew that amblyopia could be cured by covering the good eye. But there is one important condition: the occlusion must begin early enough and continue for a long enough period. There is a critical period in which amblyopia can arise and can also be cured. This period begins roughly in the first months of life and continues up to the sixth year. Vision in the first year of life is particularly vulnerable. Occlusion of an eye for a week (for instance, for an eye infection) can lead unnoticed to great loss of vision. The earlier the deprivation of visual experience starts and the longer it lasts, the deeper the amblyopia is and the more difficult it is to cure. In spite of much study, it is still not known exactly what amblyopia is. It has long been debated whether the eye has not learned to see or whether it has lost its innate power of perception. But this empiristic-nativistic alternative has been found untenable because the eye of a young child undergoes a ripening process. The development of the visual system at birth is far from complete. In the ensuing months, or even years, further growth takes place, which has largely been set on the rails already but is also modified by experience. It is therefore not surprising that the visual acuity of a new-born (which can be determined in all sorts of ingenious ways) is less than a tenth of the definitive visual acuity. In the second half of the first year of life the visual acuity has already reached a much higher level on account of the further development of the retina, but it is not until the end of the tenth year, on the completion of the cortical development, that the final result is obtained.

NEUROPHYSIOLOGY OF AMBLYOPIA

Hubel and Wiesel examined the distribution of dominance in cortical cells (Fig. 8.10), not only in adult cats but also in new-born kittens. They found the distribution

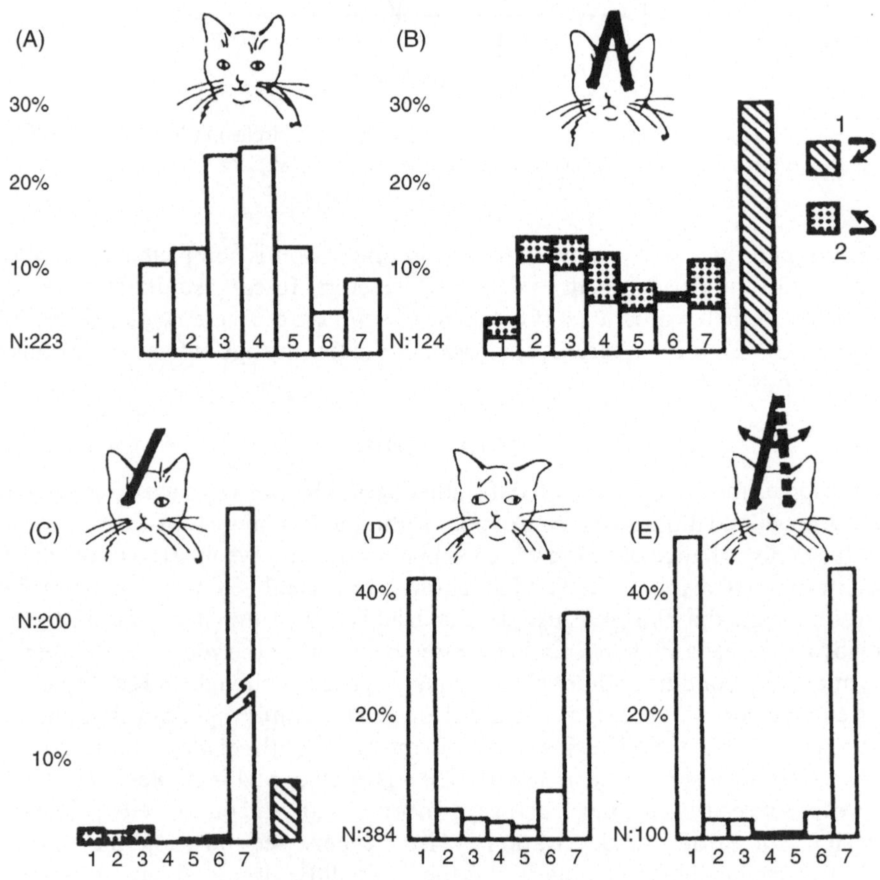

Fig. 8.10. Changes in dominance on disturbance of binocular vision. (A) Normal; (B) binocular occlusion. (1: cells without response; 2: cells without preferred orientation); (C) monocular occlusion; (D) induced divergent squint; (E) alternating occlusion.

in the kittens to be analogous to that in the adult cats, but could alter that dramatically by sewing up one of the kitten's eyes, inducing an artificial squint, or occluding the eyes alternately. Sewing up both eyes at the same time had less influence on the dominance pattern, but a large number of cells lost their ability to be stimulated and their sensitivity to orientation (Fig. 8.10). The conclusion may be drawn that (unilateral) amblyopia is based on a disturbance of equilibrium in which the good eye annexes the binocular cells, thereby not only blocking the access of the occluded eye to the cortex but also destroying binocular vision.

By sewing up one eye of kittens at various ages, the cat's sensitive period could be determined: between the third and the twelfth week. The sensitive period in the cat (and also in the ape) is thus much shorter than in man. The period in which artificial amblyopia can be induced in cats is also the period in which that amblyopia can recover if the closed eye is opened and the good eye is occluded. During this 'amblyopia treatment' the equilibrium between the right and left monocular cells is restored, but the binocular cells remain absent, as is also the case in artificially produced alternating squint. This is in agreement with clinical experience in humans.

The sensitive period has so far been described in terms of squint and amblyopia, but naturally has in the first place a physiological significance. It is assumed that the organization of the cortical connections between the cells is still being built up during the sensitive period. The cells of the newborn kitten still have weak orientation specificity and no sensitivity to disparity. Visual experience is apparently necessary for the precise attunement of the receptive fields of the binocular cells. During the period that this process has not yet been completed, binocular vision is vulnerable.

Neurophysiology has markedly deepened our insight into binocular vision, squint and amblyopia. It has become clear that the old distinction between 'innate' and 'acquired,' between nativism and empiricism, cannot be so sharply defined. For good binocular vision, subtle cooperation is needed between genetically and empirically dictated events.

It should be noted that even the most extreme amplyopia does not lead to complete blindness. It has been suggested that the 'second visual system' comes to the rescue (see p. 80) and that the amblyopic eye in this way retains a certain degree of 'ambient vision.'[3]

---

[3] Trevarthen, 1970; Crone, 1977a.

9. The Perception of Movement

INTRODUCTION

In physics, movement is a derivative: change of position per unit of time. In the psychology of the special senses, on the other hand, movement is a primary perceptual fact, as real as position. That signifies that in our spatial vision, movement is possible without change of position and change of position is possible without movement.

Just as many special senses give us information about the spatial position of ourselves and our surroundings, that also applies to our and their movements. Rest and movement are not only decided by the eye, but also by the touch and the organ of equilibrium. Luckily these decisions are seldom conflicting. When that is the case we become bewildered. When a 3D film takes us on a switchback at a dizzy speed, we experience no changes in the pressure of our bodies on the cinema seat and our organs of equilibrium remain unstimulated. The conflict between information from various movement-sensitive senses makes us nauseous. The subjective space which is determined by more than one of our senses loses its stability. The same thing happens when the organ of equilibrium gives us information which is not confirmed by our organs of sight. It is well known that people become more easily seasick in a cabin than on deck. That is not only because the air is fresher but also, and mainly, because the visual stimuli are then in agreement with the stimuli from the vestibule. In the discussion of the visual sense of movement, this sort of multimodal sensory phenomenon will be avoided as far as possible. It is not completely possible, because visual space is embedded in the space which is built up by various special senses together, and is therefore difficult to understand in strict isolation.

THREE FORMS OF MOVEMENT PERCEPTION

Movement can be seen in three different circumstances. In the first place, a moving object can be seen with a stationary eye. Secondly, the movement of an object can be seen that is fixated at the fovea and is being followed by the eye. And finally, there is movement perception that is not activated by movement in physical space but is still dependent on visual mechanisms: apparent movement.

MOVEMENT PERCEPTION WITH A STATIONARY EYE

A visible movement has a direction, a position in the visual field, and a velocity. In everyday life naturally movements take place in all directions, but the research worker has an understandable preference for movements in the fronto-parallel plane. Movements in the direction of gaze are more difficult to analyse. When a car comes from a distance directly towards us, it gets steadily bigger. The contours of the car do not all move in one direction, like in movements in the frontal plane, but in all directions at the same time.

A movement can be seen in the outer periphery of the visual field, but also close to the fixation point. The sensitivity to the movement of small objects is greatest at the centre of the visual field. Just as with directional and depth perception, there is in movement perception also a difference between absolute and relative thresholds. The relative threshold of the visible movement of an object against a structured background is low; it is usually said to be one minute of arc per second. We only need to look at our watches to see that there is a limit to our perception of movement: we see the second-hand moving but not the minute-hand. The absolute threshold, the visibility of a moving point of light in a dark room, is about ten times as high. That may cause surprise, because in directional and stereoscopic vision the difference betwee absolute and relative thresholds is so much greater. The explanation lies in the fact that absolute immobility does not exist for the visual system. There is *autokinesis*, a phenomenon that will be considered in the section on apparent movement.

In the periphery of the visual field the sensitivity for large moving objects is greater than for stationary objects. In the extreme periphery only moving stimuli are seen (Fig. 9.1). The relatively high sensitivity for movement in the periphery has an obvious biological function. The peripheral retina is specialised in the detection of danger, i.e., movement.

There is also an upper threshold for movement perception. We see a wasp fly, but not a bullet. Above a velocity of about thirty degrees per second the perception of

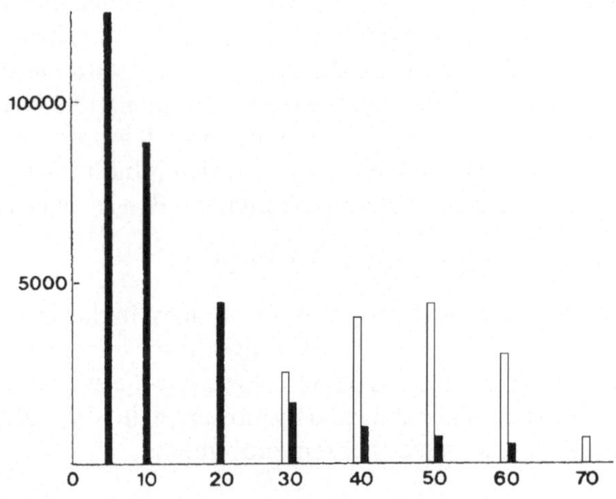

Fig. 9.1. Sensitivity of the retinal periphery to movement. Number of stationary (black bars) and moving (white bars) image elements distinguishable in concentric, 1-degree wide, circles of the visual field (Crone, 1977b).

vision begins to fail. Large objects are still seen to move at much greater angular velocities.

MOVEMENT PERCEPTION WITH THE FOLLOWING EYE

A moving object can be fixated on the fovea centralis by a gliding movement of the eye, a 'following movement,' and even so still be seen to be moving. Following movements have a specific character that differs in many ways from saccades. While saccades are rapid ballistic movements, the direction and velocity of which cannot be changed in midstream, following movements are slower and their direction and velocity can be altered. While the adequate stimulus for a saccade is the *position* of a peripheral retinal stimulus, the adequate stimulus for the start of a following movement is the *direction* and the *velocity* of a local retinal stimulus. A stationary stimulus on the retina can only in special circumstances lead to a following movement, as will be seen in the next section.

Following movements and saccades have a very important property in common. They are both non-reflex and *intentional*; they do not disturb the stability of subjective space. Again we encounter the 'equivalence principle.' In earlier chapters it was in connection with the equivalence of directional vision by means of peripheral local signs and of gaze innervation, and the equivalence of depth perception by means of disparity and convergence. Now, in the case of movement perception, it is the equivalence of movement over the retina and following movements. Let us not worry our heads too much about why the world stays still during intentional eye movements. It is a basic element of our knowledge, about which physiology can teach us little (see p. 59).

FOLLOWING MOVEMENTS AND PARAFOVEAL FIXATION

A parafoveal stimulus which does not move over the retina may give rise to a following movement. Some people have so-called 'mouches volantes,' small opacities in the vitreous, which are seen as small flies in the visual field if they are close to the retina. If one sees a mouche volante just to the right of the direction of fixation, one is inclined to try and fixate it. But that attempt has no success: the eye makes a following movement to the right but the distance from the fixation point remains the same. If one flashes with a camera to the right of the fixation point, an after-image is produced that it is useless to try and fixate. In this case also, the eyes make a following movement to the right without being able to reach the after-image. Extremely precise investigation of after-images shows that there is a relationship between the velocity of the following movement and the distance between the after-image and the centre of fixation.

The question arises, how close is the connection between the following movement and the parafoveal fixation. In the above cases the following movement is the *result* of parafoveal stimulation. But is the reverse a possibility: that the following movement is the *cause* of parafoveal stimulation? That has been found to be possible, as shown in Figure 9.2. When the eye is forced to make a following movement (fixation of a light source through a rotating prism), the (mean) fixation shifts in the parafoveal direction.

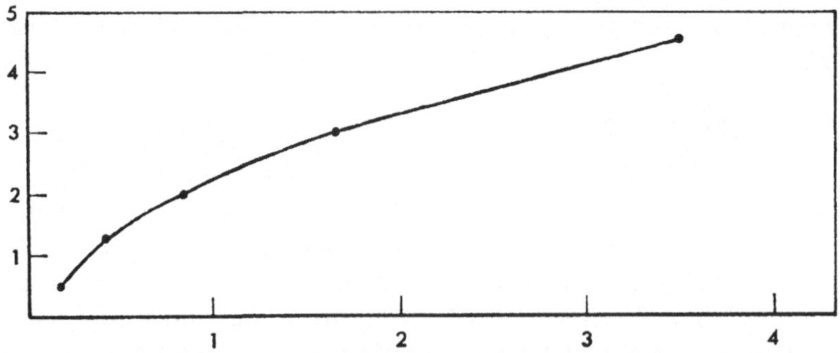

Fig. 9.2. The lag of the eye during pursuit. Abscissa: mean velocity of target (degrees per second); ordinate: mean eccentricity of fixation (minutes of arc) (Crone & Verduyn Lunel, 1969).

One might ask oneself how the eye knows, when it is fixating a moving aeroplane in a cloudless sky, that it must continue the following movement? There are two answers. Firstly, everyone knows that an aeroplane in the air cannot suddenly stand still. The continuation of the following movement has a predictive character and is thus centrally determined. But Figure 8.2 also teaches us that the following movement can be maintained by a peripheral stimulus: the parafoveal fixation.

APPARENT MOVEMENT

WANDERING STARS

In 1799, when the famous explorer, Alexander von Humboldt, climbed the volcano in Teneriffe before daybreak, he saw a low-lying star move. He presumed that it was a curious atmospheric phenomenon. His conviction was supported by the fact that Prince Adalbert of Prussia had seen the same thing at the same place fifty years earlier. It soon became apparent, however, that the drifting of a point of light in the dark was quite common, and not limited to the Canary Islands and aristocratic observers. A German physiologist, whose classical education had not been wasted, called the phenomenon 'autokinesis,' the word used by Plato to describe the movement of the soul, in its carriage drawn by winged but unruly horses.

The drifting movement of a point of light in the dark is found to be due to unstable (mean) fixation. In an experiment (Fig. 9.3), in which a small point of light is fixated in the dark, and the installation is such that an illuminated new moon appears on the side to which the fixation has drifted, it is seen that the apparent movement nearly always takes place in the opposite direction (away from the concave side of the moon). Autokinesis to the right apparently occurs when the mean direction of gaze drifts slightly to the left of the point of light. The connection between parafoveal fixation and the perception of movement was mentioned above, and is again clear in autokinesis. Autokinesis is a slow movement, less than 15 minutes of arc per second, and thus lies below the threshold of real absolute movement. The remarkable feature of autokinesis is that one sees movement

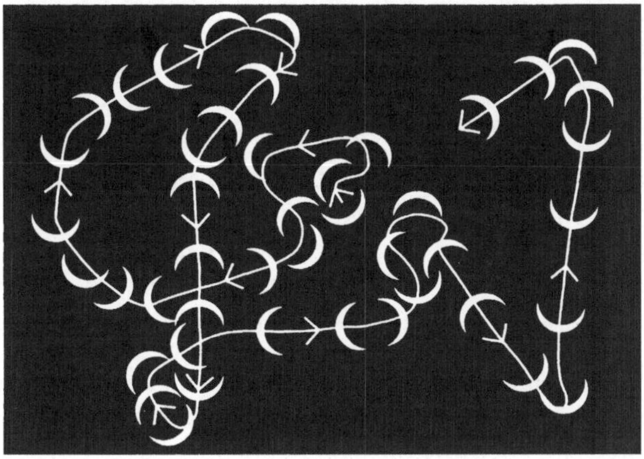

Fig. 9.3. A light fixated in the dark appears to move as shown by the white line. A signal is flashed at regular intervals with which a new moon is seen if the fixation is not precisely centred. The new moon is seen on the side towards which the fixation has drifted. The apparent movement is in the opposite direction (Crone & Verduyn Lunel, 1969).

without displacement. This emphasizes the fact once more that movement is a visual quality in its own right, not derived from the visual direction.

INDUCED MOVEMENT

A bird that is flying between trees is moving, and the trees are standing still. There can be no doubt about that. In other instances it is not so clear what is moving and what is standing still. At a station, from your own carriage when you can only see the train next to you, you can well imagine that train has begun to move slowly when in actual fact it is your own train that has started to move. This optical illusion is called 'induced movement.' When large objects move relative to small objects, the illusion is much stronger. At night the moon can suddenly be seen to appear from behind a large cloud. The illusion of a moving moon is compulsive.

THE WATERFALL ILLUSION

When an English psychologist in 1834 sat day-dreaming on the banks of Loch Ness, he stared for a long time at the tumbling water of a waterfall. When he finally turned his eyes away he saw the surrounding rocks moving upwards. This phenomenon could be explained as follows: When an object is at rest in the vertical direction, there is equilibrium between the resting activities of perceptive elements sensitive to upward and downward movements. When one looks at a waterfall for a long time, the receptors for downward movement become exhausted (adapted). If one then looks at the rocks beside the waterfall, the resting activity of the receptors for upward movement is temporarily dominant. It will become clear when the neurophysiology of movement perception is considered, that this explanation is well founded. The motion after-effect plays an important part in the psychological investigation of movement perception.

THE FILM

When in an experiment time and distance are well chosen, it makes no difference to our sensation whether a point of light moves from A to B, or the light at A goes out and the light at B goes on. This phenomenon, called by psychologists the phi-phenomenon, is one of the two pillars on which film is based. In reality, nothing moves over the screen in the cinema, but a rapid succession of stationary images are presented. The other pillar is the 'retinal slowness' (Charpentier, 1886). Even an image that is presented extremely shortly has subjectively a certain duration. When children play with sparklers at Christmas and make circles in the air, they see an illuminated ring, because the light impression has not died out in the time that the sparkler has made a complete circle.

THE NEUROPHYSIOLOGY OF MOVEMENT PERCEPTION

The neurophysiology of the perception of movement begins in the retina. In the retinas of rabbits ganglion cells have been found which are specifically sensitive to movement over the retina in a certain direction. This does not apply to apes, but it may be presumed that it is principally the alpha-cells of the retina which are responsible for the perception of movement. These project onto the magnocellular layer in the LGN, which is concerned with movement.

New insights suggest that there are at least two channels, one for higher speeds and one for lower. They run separately in the cerebrum. The channel for slower movements may play a part in the recognition of objects. Many objects which are held in the hand are easier to recognize if they are turned in various directions.

When we considered the neurophysiology of the visual acuity, we already mentioned that many cells in area V1 are sensitive to the orientation of the stimulus. But those cells are also sensitive to the direction of movement of the stimulus (Fig. 9.4). The posterior part of the parietal lobe and the middle temporal area MT (area V5) are the higher visual centres which contribute most to the control of following movements. From these areas and the frontal ocular fields efferent nerves go to the brain stem. The details are not known, but in view of the close relationship between the following movements and the slow phase of optokinetic nystagmus, it seems probable that these two types of movement finally have a common path.

THE PATHOLOGY OF MOVEMENT PERCEPTION

As stated in this chapter, movement perception is a separate modality of vision, with its own neurones in the visual cortex and its own higher centres in the temporal, parietal and frontal lobes. But in occipito-parietal and occipito-temporal lesions it is usually the case that visuo-spatial and visuo-motor outfall symptoms occur together. The clinician then often sees a hemianopia with outfall of following movements, so that a moving object is followed by means of a series of saccades. Patients with an isolated disturbance of movement perception are seldom seen.

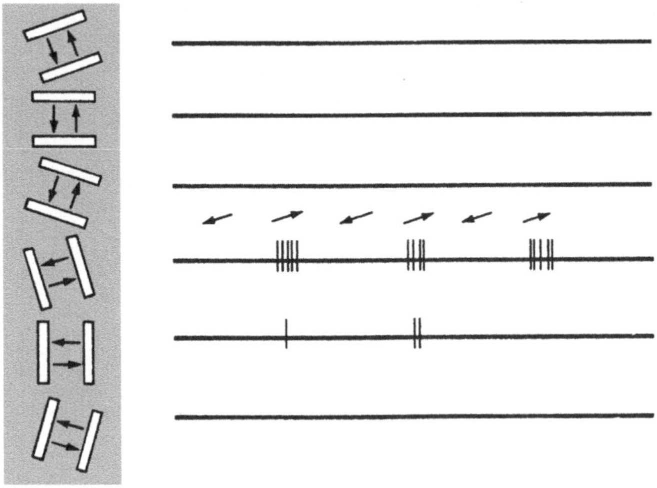

Fig. 9.4. A movement- and orientation-sensitive cell. This cell responds exclusively to a slit moving upwards and to the right in the eleven o'clock orientation (Hubel & Wiesel, 1958).

A patient who probably had a bilateral lesion of the MT area, saw a passing car change position but did not see it move. It was bewildering for this patient to move in a crowd, because the people didn't stream backwards as she walked passed them, as happens with normal movement perception[1]. Slow movements can sometimes be recognized by such patients; yet another proof that the neural tracts for fast and slow movements run separate courses.

[1] Grüsser and Landis, 1991.

10. Theories of the Visual Perception of Space

INTRODUCTION

On p. 14 it was explained that spatial behaviour must be seen biologically as a sensorimotor process. But when studying human beings, attention can also be paid to the subjective perception of space. When a man sees a ripe apple hanging in a tree and picks it, a sensorimotor process takes place that begins in the retina and results in movement, but at the same time there is the perception of the apple and the consciousness that one wants to pick it. *But what if one doesn't want to pick the apple*? Then seeing the apple in space is all that remains and one tends to forget the possibility of a motor intention. In this way, the psychological point of view becomes alienated from the biological, which nevertheless has priority in the existing hierarchy.

The *psychological* analysis of spatial vision, which disregards the biological aspects of vision as a sensorimotor process, has a long history. This history began with the Greeks, but survived tenaciously until the last century.

A *sensorimotor* analysis of spatial vision is of later date, when Descartes laid the foundations of modern, materialistic physiology. He had few followers until neurophysiology blossomed in the 20th century, and the path from retinal stimulus to motor effect could slowly be traced.

THE PSYCHOLOGICAL THEORY OF SPATIAL VISION IN HISTORICAL PERSPECTIVE[1]

The Greeks, who were just beginning to study vision, realized that looking was a mental activity. They thought that the eyes sent out 'visual rays,' with which they scanned the outside world. It was a natural train of thought: a man looks out for danger, searches with his eyes, gives something a glance. Of course the Greeks had no idea of the physical properties of rays but, in view of their interest in geometry, the idea of something coming out of the eye in a straight line was attractive. An important argument in favour of the 'extramission theory' of vision was that eyes could radiate 'fire.' This could be best seen in cats. It was one of the most tenacious misconceptions. In 1700 Bidloo, a professor of medicine in Leyden, performed the

[1] van Hoorn, 1972; Lindberg, 1976.

'cat test' (Bidloo, 1715). He shut himself up, together with a cat, in a completely dark room. When they both came out again, the professor declared positively that in complete darkness no light came out of the cat's eyes! Incidentally, with this statement Bidloo declared himself in disagreement with no-one less than Descartes, at that time an authoritative philosopher.

But even for the Greeks the extramission theory had one weak point: the light. Light plays a predominant role in vision. But light comes from the sun and not from the eye. For this reason Democritus was an intromissionist. He thought that vision was a sort of contact with images, *eidola*, material emanations of things. Lucretius, the Roman poet and follower of Democritus, speaks later of *simulacra*, and compares these with the discarded skin of a snake. Aristotle was also an intramissionist; he thought that the eye was specifically sensitive to colour. For definitive perception he thought that other, less specific, information was necessary, such as shape, movement and likeness to other objects. Apparently Aristotle considered colour to be the 'primary quality' and space a 'secondary quality.' It was not until Aristotelism had fallen during the scientific revolution, that Locke began to call colour secondary and space primary!

Euclid (300 BC), the great mathematician, was the first to show explicit interest in spatial vision. He gave the first impulse to the theory of perspective. He explained on geometrical grounds why a tree in the distance appeared smaller than one nearby and why a circle appears as a line when it is lying in the plane of the eye. Euclid thought in terms of visual rays that diverged as a cone in straight lines from the eye. Ptolemy (150 AD, thus 400 years later), the astronomer, also studied light and vision. Greek optics reached its summit in his work. His most important findings regarding binocular vision have been mentioned on p. 87.

Ibn al Haytham (1000, Alhazen) is the first to practise physiological optics. Like Aristotle he takes the view that vision is a passive occurrence. Instead of the latter's holistic conception of shape he introduces the atomistic idea of light-radiating points. But he takes a further, crucial step: he propounds the idea that every point in the outside world is represented on the lens, which is the real organ of sight. With this theory, optics enters the eye for the first time, and one can speak of an 'image' of the outside world in the eye. That image is the right way up (Fig. 10.1). Alhazen's book on optics was translated into Latin with the title *Perspectiva*. It became the source of inspiration for the mediaeval students of optics, who are still called the 'perspectivists.' Important perspectivists were Roger Bacon and Witelo (Vitellio), who both lived around 1250. Bacon accepted Alhazen's theory, but could not completely reject the idea of extramission: in addition to the power of the light rays which come towards us, a power goes out in the opposite direction.

JOHANNES KEPLER AND THE PROJECTION THEORY

Science was not advancing swiftly at that time; in 1572 the optical works of Witelo were printed, in one volume with Alhazen's work, under the title *Opticae thesaurus*. Shortly afterwards, in 1604, the astronomer Johannes Kepler wrote his 'corollary to Witelo's work' (*Ad Vitellionem paralipomena*), in which he suggested that the outside world is not represented the right way up on the lens but upside down on the

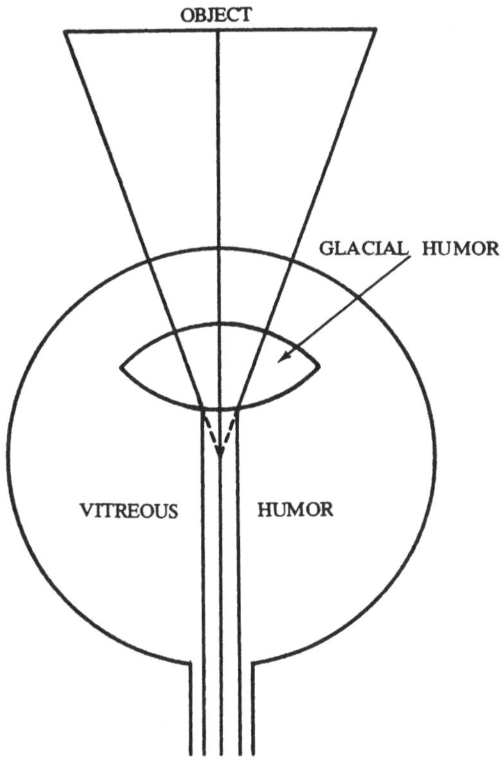

Fig. 10.1. The geometry of sight according to Alhazen (1000). All points of the object emits rays in many directions, but only the rays that are perpendicular to the cornea, contribute to the image (after Lindberg, 1976).

retina. It was the most important discovery ever made in physiological optics, but confronted the psychology of spatial vision with almost insoluble problems.

Kepler's theory of the inverted retinal image (Fig. 10.2) was difficult to reconcile with established opinions. His theory conflicted with that of Aristotle and many scholars of the time. According to them, the 'shapes,' realistic images of the outside world, forced their way into the senses. In such a theory, an inverted retinal image must lead to a world seen upside down.

An attempt to solve this problem was made by assuming that the soul, which sees the retinal image from the inside, turns it right side up again. But the hypothesis of a *homunculus*, a little man in your head, stranded. Because who provides the retinal image with the homunculus? If one thinks about it, one sees a succession of steadily smaller homunculi, like Russian dolls that fit into each other.

Kepler himself had a different solution (Fig. 10.3). The mental lines from the retina to the outside world follow the same path as the rays travelling inwards, so that the inversion is abolished. This is the famous 'projection theory.' This explanation was also doomed to fail because it involved visual rays that were not in agreement with modern ideas.

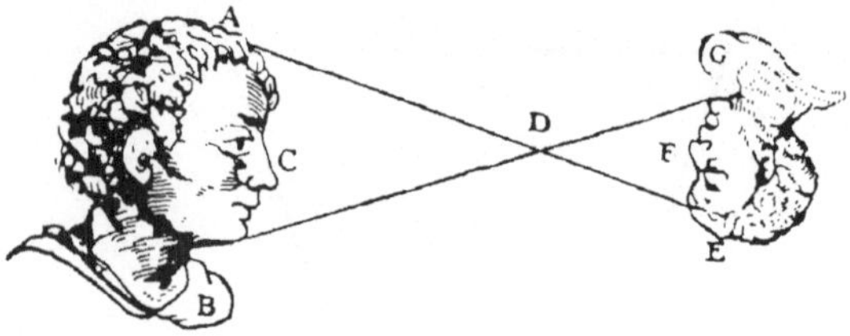

Fig. 10.2. The inverted retinal image (after Descartes, 1637).

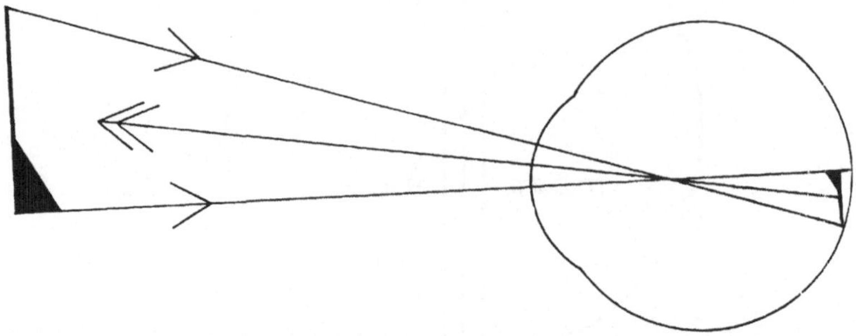

Fig. 10.3. Kepler's projection theory. The inverted retinal image is projected into space in the upright position.

The psychological theory of spatial vision which, with one small step (the retina), had placed itself outside its own territory, clung anxiously to the idea that the visual process was a retinal process, although it was known that the eyes were connected with the brain by the optic nerves and that the brain was therefore presumably involved in vision. Kepler himself thought that 'sight itself descends from the high court of the brain to the optic nerve and the retina, as if they were lower courts of justice, and there meets the image on the retina.'

In spite of the progressive advance of the natural sciences, most people continued to see vision as a retinal function. The German brain-anatomist Reil translated Kepler's theory two centuries later into anatomical terms. He thought (1795) that visual images were presented diffusely in the brain and were finally led back to the optic nerves. The physiologist Johannes Müller, as ignorant as Kepler and Reil of the precise cerebral representation of vision, was in agreement with this theory (1840). He spoke of the 'Selbstanschauung der Netzhaut' (self-observation of the retina).

The problem of the inverted retinal image continued to disturb numerous scholars. As previously mentioned (p. 22), Buffon thought that newborns at first saw everything upside down, until the moment that visual space, with the help of experiences gained by touch, was turned right way up. Donders too, the famous author of *On the Anomalies of Accommodation and Refraction in the Eye* (1864), had something similar in mind: 'Through this double inversion,' he says in the

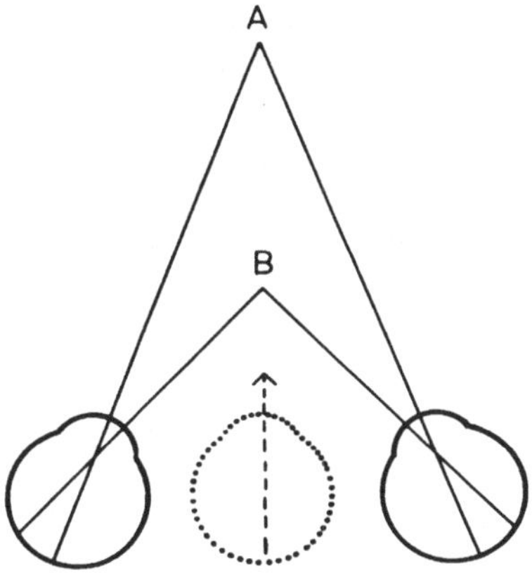

Fig. 10.4. The cyclopean eye.

introduction to his refraction theory,'the projected image corresponds to the object, although, properly speaking, only the projected retinal image stands, as it were, before our eyes.' Lines from the psyche enter the retina and run from there to the object. The realization that the image of the outside world was a mental image although the brain belonged to the material world, was still beyond anyone's conception.

The projection theory is still alive in the minds of many ophthalmologists and practitioners of physiological optics today. In the theory of squint, for instance, psychic lines are still drawn leaving an imaginary eye. That imaginary eye is the so-called 'cyclopean eye.' The German physiologists Helmholtz and Hering realized that binocular vision was a problem for the projection theory. When a nearby object is seen, the fixated object lies to the right in the left eye and to the left in the right eye. With the cyclopean eye, a combination of the two real eyes, the problem was solved (Fig. 10.4). By means of an artifice, the binocular image could still be projected outwards in an orderly fashion.

THE SENSORIMOTOR THEORY OF SPATIAL VISION IN HISTORICAL PERSPECTIVE[2]

DESCARTES

The inverted retinal image demanded a new theory of vision. This was provided by the most important theorist at the time of the scientific revolution: René Descartes. He is the central figure at the transition from mediaeval scholasticism to modern natural science.

Descartes' theory of vision is mechanistic (Fig. 4.19). The fibres of the optic nerves, which run separately even in the chiasma, transmit the mechanical disturbances brought about by light in the retina. The fibres work as stretched strings: if one end is pulled it has an effect at the other end. In this way a twofold representation

[2] Descartes, 1664; Lotze, 1852; Roelofs, 1935, 1960; Crone, 1973, 1988.

of the outside world develops in the brain, one from each eye. With the help of animal spirits present in the brain cavities, the information from both representations is combined in the *sensorium commune.*

Although, in this process, none of the information that was present in the retina is lost, the internal representation only slightly resembles what was actually seen. The cerebral picture is different from the outside world, it is in many ways contra-intuitive; as we should say now: coded. Descartes says (1637) the following about the cerebral images: 'They only need to resemble the objects in a couple of ways, and their perfection is often dependent on the degree to which they do not so strongly resemble the things as they might; it is, take note, only important how the images enable the spirit to observe all the various properties of things, not how much the images resemble the things themselves.' It is a surprisingly modern observation.

In animals, creatures without a soul, the cerebral visual signals are integrated in the *sensorium commune* with signals from other special senses and information from the memory (Descartes localised the 'physical memory' in the convolutions of the brain). After the above process of integration and association, an impulse goes from the brain to the muscles. In human beings, blessed with a soul, signals which have been decoded in the pineal body are deciphered by the soul and translated into sensory perceptions. There, certain mechanical whirls become colour, others become sound. Descartes does not try to deduce the perceptions from the mechanical occurrence: these are creations of God's Providence.

In this way, Descartes describes the pathway from a sensory organ via the brain to an effector organ (Fig. 10.5). In the drawing he shows how a woman points her finger at an arrow; he might just as well have drawn a cat stretching out a claw to a mouse.

LOTZE

Descartes' physiological concept of spatial vision received little attention in the next two centuries. Everyone was too much occupied with psychology. It is to the credit of Rudolph Hermann Lotze (1817–1881) that Descartes' physiological theory reappeared. Lotze, who has studied philosophy and medicine, tries to combine physiological and psychological facts into one coherent system. At the age of thirty-five he writes his *Medizinische Psychologie* (1852) with the significant subtitle 'or, physiology of the soul' (*oder Physiologie der Seele*). In this book he examines the course of the sensorimotor process, 'which, from the reception of external impressions, through manifold inner processing, leads to movements and acts.' In this sense, he also tackles the spatial problem.

Lotze's spatial theory is known as the theory of 'local signs.' Retinal elements do not only give a colour signal, but also a spatial signal. The local sign can be compared to the postal code, that shows the destination of a letter. All the letters come together at a zero point, the non-spatial soul. That is where the letters are sorted. After that they fan out to their destinations. *For the local signs, the destinations are the eye muscles, through which the eye is directed towards the object*. But spatial localisation does not only take place through *movement* of the eye; when a peripheral point in the

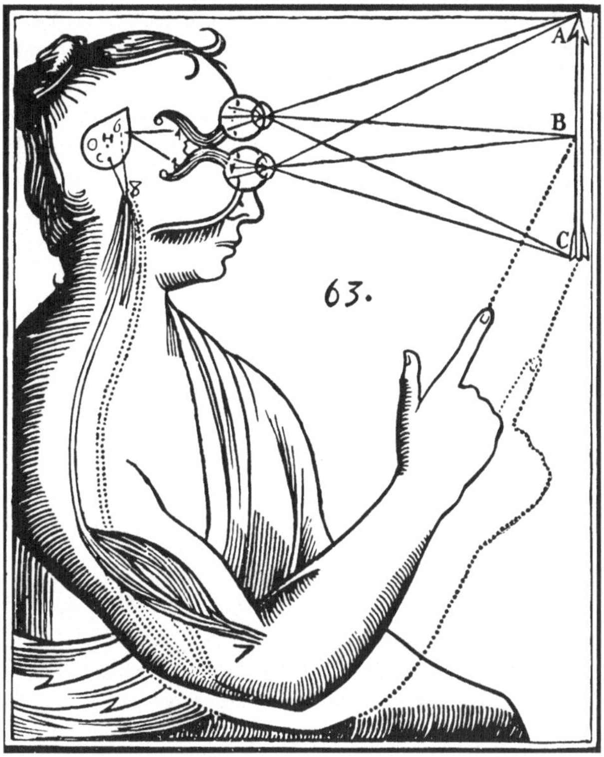

Fig. 10.5. Visual localisation according to Descartes (1664). The visual stimulus directs the pointing finger via central nervous connections.

retina is stimulated, an eye movement may be made, but it is also possible that it does not take place. In the latter case, only an intention to move, a '*Bewegungstrieb*' is produced in the nervous system, which itself sends a signal for localisation.

Lotze thinks on Cartesian lines. He considers that a geometrical representation of space in the nervous system is not necessary. That signifies that he approaches spatial localisation as a kind of information processing, for which a picture-in-the-head is not needed. The theory goes a step further in the crucial role given to the eye movements, whether these are effectuated or not.

Lotze's theory attracted few followers at the time. There were three, more or less minor, weak points in his theory, which made it easy for his critics. There was his empiristic viewpoint, which was gradually becoming less popular. Lotze thought that the relationship between the strength of the eye movements and the extent of the local signs had to be learnt. In addition, Lotze thought that localisation was based on the registration of feelings of tension signed back by the eye muscles. Helmholtz later demonstrated decisively that sensations in the eye muscles played no important part in localisation. But the main reason why Lotze's theory was not accepted was that his contemporaries could not free themselves of the projection theory and a purely psychological analysis of spatial perception.

Lotze's thesis that visual perception of space must be viewed as a sensorimotor process is certainly correct. But someone who asks himself how a cat catches a mouse does not think in the first place of eye movements. The fact that Lotze did think like that demonstrates deep insight and, at the same time, a sensible limitation. The deep insight refers to the fact that the eye muscles undoubtedly are at the bottom of all visually-controlled movement. The sensible limitation was correct because there was complete lack of any knowledge of the course of impulses from the retinal local signs to the motor system of the body. The pathway from the local signs to the eye muscles is complicated enough in itself.

ROELOFS AND THE PRINCIPLE OF EQUIVALENCE

In 1935 and 1960, Roelofs, long ago my teacher, wrote important studies on the physiological aspects of spatial vision. He accepted much of Lotze's theory, but not his empiricism or his hypothesis about the muscle sensitivity of the eye muscles. On the basis of many arguments (too many to be listed in this book), he demonstrated that optical localisation of position, movement and depth can be equated with the nervous stimulation of an eye muscle which, when effected, leads to eye movement and, when not carried out, produces a tension pattern that is of equal value for localisation. Every spatial point that we see owes its position to the stimulus, *or the invitation*, to an eye movement.

This is the 'equivalence theory,' which has been elaborated in the previous chapters. (1) Directional localisation is achieved in two ways, either by a gaze movement, which annuls the local sign, or by the local sign itself, which creates tension when the gaze impulse is not put into effect. (2) The localisation of movement also comes about in two ways, either by a following movement which annuls the movement of the retinal image, or by the movement of the retinal image itself, creating tension if the following movement is not carried out. (3) For depth localisation the situation is analogous. It results either from a vergence movement which annuls the local sign (the binocular disparity), or from the disparity itself, when the impulse to vergence is not effectuated.

STABILITY AND PLASTICITY OF VISUAL ORIENTATION

The physiological theory of space presumes a fixed relationship between the stimulation of the retina and the movement of the eye. In lower animals this is the case. In the forties Sperry and Stone rotated the eyes of salamanders through 180 degrees. The motor responses of the animals to light stimuli remained subsequently in the opposite direction to the stimulus (Fig. 10.6). Hess's experiments (1956) also demonstrated the marked stability of the retinal local signs. Hess put small rubber caps fitted with prisms (base outwards) over the heads of newborn chicks, thus producing over-convergence of the eyes. This made them peck in front of the grains in their feed (Fig. 10.7) Even long practice did not enable them to overcome this motor error.

These facts need not surprise us. In the previous pages the idea has been developed that our behaviour in visual space is determined by motor impulses which arise in the retina and generate—effectuated or not effectuated—eye movements. It is a fundamental process which must be unshakably established in our organism.

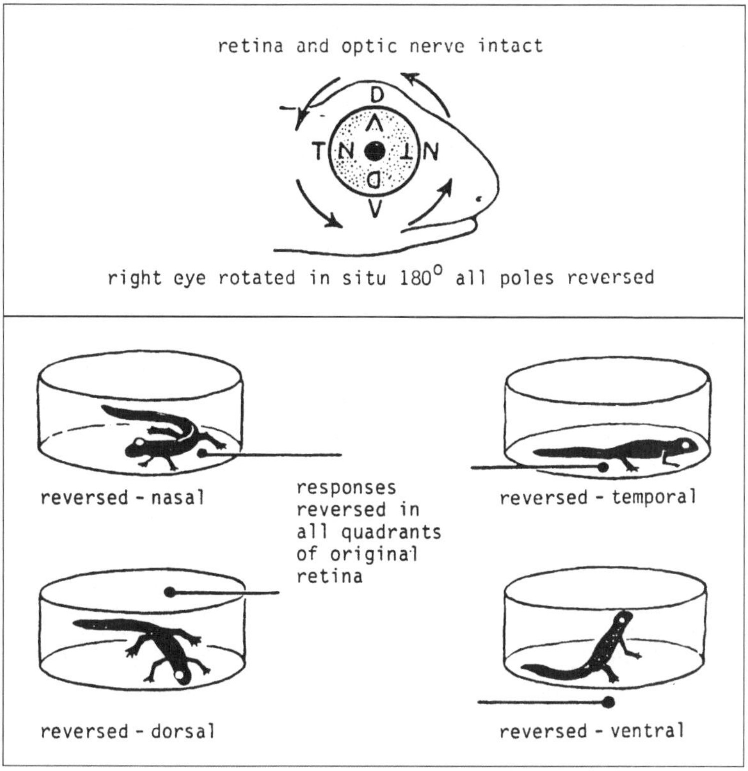

Fig. 10.6. Reversed motor reactions of salamander after rotation of the eye through 180 degrees (Stone, 1947).

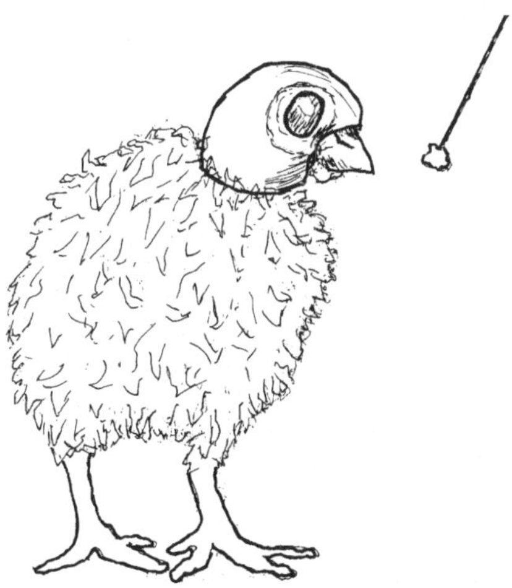

Fig. 10.7. Innate stereoscopic vision (Hess, 1956). Chickens with prisma glasses that make the rays of light converge, peck in front of the offered grains.

This viewpoint is diametrically opposed to that of the English empiricists, who thought that the mind was a *tabula rasa*, a clean slate, to be written on by experience. Helmholtz too, strongly influenced by John Locke, thought that the relation between the local sign and the motor impulse was calibrated by experience. However, on the grounds of numerous facts, everyone is now convinced that organisms develop according to fixed laws, laid down in the genes, although a certain amount of modification is possible through practising and learning.

The experiments performed by the American psychologist Stratton (1896) spread doubts and confusion in this field. Stratton tried to solve an old problem. Why do we see objects the right side up when the retinal image is upside down? We must have had to learn to adjust our movements to the inverted position of the retinal image. Being a convinced empiricist, he thought that we would be able to overcome this adjustment if the retinal image was turned right side up by an inverting optic system. In his remarkable experiment he wore for a number of days a keplerian telescope with magnification 1:1 in front of one eye and kept the other eye occluded. At first everything seemed completely abnormal. He saw the visual world upside down. If he saw something on the right he tried to grasp it with his right hand, but discovered that he should have used his left hand. Gradually he began to control his movements better and sometimes the world seemed to be right way up again. Stratton's experiment has been repeated many times and the results are controversial. Some authors agreed that the world became the right way up, thus proving the doctrine of the old empiricists that the touch is the teacher of vision. Others declared the opposite, and stated that vision is the teacher of touch and the kinetic sense.

An enormous amount of literature has been produced on the problem of the reorganisation of visual space, but an important point has nearly always been overlooked: no reorganisation has taken place between the retinal local sign and the eye movements. Someone who looks through an inverting telescope sees more or less the same as the early photographer, who looked from under his black cloth at the inverted image on the frosted glass. He knows that the image is inverted, but can allow his eyes to travel unhindered over that image: *the relationship between local sign and eye movement is not inverted.* That inversion was accomplished in 1970 by K.U. Smith using a complicated electronic technique. In such an experiment the eye movement is registered and the inverted registration is yoked to the position of a fixation point on a screen. Under these conditions, when a fixation movement is made to the right the fixation point on the screen jumps to the left. Test persons could not adjust to such a bewildering inversion, which made the visual field unstable and jittery. Stratton and his followers proved that a learning process could lead to far-reaching adjustments between vision and body movement, but the fundamental physiological concept that the local sign in the retina and the eye movement are one, still remains standing.

And what about the relationship between the biretinal local sign and the vergence? Another computer program was devised (Schmidt et al., 1974), to yoke the fixation point the wrong way round to the convergent and divergent movements of the eye. Convergent movements made the fixation point appear further away to the observer, while divergence had the opposite effect. The reversal of the vergence movements causes binocular vision to degenerate to random fixation movements at various distances. There was little or no adaptation to the reversal of the vergence relative to the disparity. We may thus conclude that traditional research into reversed or otherwise displaced vision has not threatened, in the long run, the sensorimotor theory of space perception. In fact, Smith and his co-workers draw the conclusion that 'the evolution of the retinal and brain mechanisms has proceeded in relation to the imperatives for dynamic direction-specific control of retinal images by lateral and vergence movements of the eyes.'

THE FUTURE OF A SENSORIMOTOR THEORY OF SPATIAL LOCALISATION

Roelofs was aware of the fact that eye movements are only the beginning of spatial localisation. Let us take another look at Descartes' drawing (Fig. 10.5). The question of how the finger is pointed remains unanswered. It may be true that the first stage of visual localisation is achieved by eye movements, but the final goal is movement of the body, the hands and the feet. For this purpose, the eyes must be coupled with other motor and sensory control systems.

An example of coordination between the senses is the control of the head and eyes by the visual sense and the sense of equilibrium. The head moves together with the gaze movements. It makes no difference to the localisation of a visual object whether the eyes are directed towards it or the head. The coupling of the eyes and the head via the organ of equilibrium takes place quite differently. The organ of equilibrium controls the eyes in such a way that the eyes make a countermovement to every movement of the head, thus guaranteeing the stability of the outside world on the retina. The organ of equilibrium thus produces countermovements of the eyes and head, while the gaze impulse produces movements in the same direction. Both systems are highly coordinated; they make use of the same switchboard for eye movements, but in a different manner. The system of eye movements must also be coordinated with the motor system of the hand, which is under the influence of vision, touch and kinaesthesia. That demands a complete hierarchy of, as yet largely unknown, topographical charts in the cerebrum.

PART III: Identification of Objects in Space

11. Contours and Surfaces

INTRODUCTION

In the previous pages I have considered the main elements of spatial vision: directions, movements, stereoscopic distances. We haven't got very far that way. Intuitively we all know what sight is for: to be able, with the help of light, to observe, identify and localise the things in the world. But we haven't even got that far. It almost seems as if our real purpose: to understand vision better, gets further away as we try to get nearer to it. To use a musical metaphor: it seems as though so far we've only been occupied with pitch, tone and the position of the players in the orchestra, but haven't yet paid any attention to the melody, the composition.

Early investigators also realized how difficult it was to get past the visual elements to the things themselves. Locke and Helmholtz both expressed opinions about this. Helmholtz thought that perception arose from elementary data such as light, colour, position and movement, and that recognition of objects was based on experience: every new observation calls up memories of previous visual experiences. By means of subconscious inferences, these experiences contribute to the perception and identification of objects.

The theory of the construction of perceptions out of sensory elements, assembled with the help of associations and subconscious inferences, fitted into the scientific atmosphere of the period. Matter consisted of a collection of atoms, observation consisted of a collection of primary sensations.

At the same time, there was a countermovement in Germany: in opposition to Helmholtz' 'atomism,' there was still the 'holism' of the idealists, Hegel's thesis that the whole had precedence over the component parts. At the beginning of the nineteenth century a holistic wave flooded sensory psychology. A group of psychologists attacked 'atomism' in psychology and turned demonstratively to the whole. These 'Gestalt psychologists' studied configurations, forms, patterns, and their movements. They had good arguments for this. One of these was the 'constancy' of visual objects: if somebody walks towards us we don't see him getting bigger; the 'Gestalt,' the configuration, stays the same, although it is continually built up of different, more widely spaced, retinal information. Gestalt psychology gave rise to a whole series of laws which are basic to the organization of form: laws of group formation (on the basis of mutual proximity and similarity) and of classification into figure and background (on the basis of closed contours, etc.). Numerous experiments

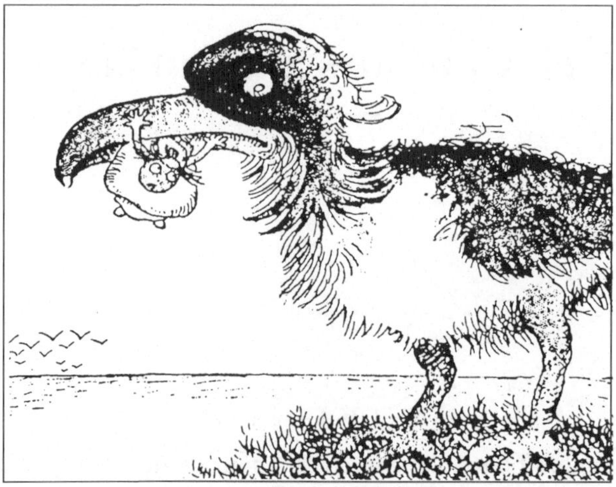

Fig. 11.1. Vision is the interpretation of figures. This picture by Gustave Verbeek shows something quite different when it is viewed upside down.

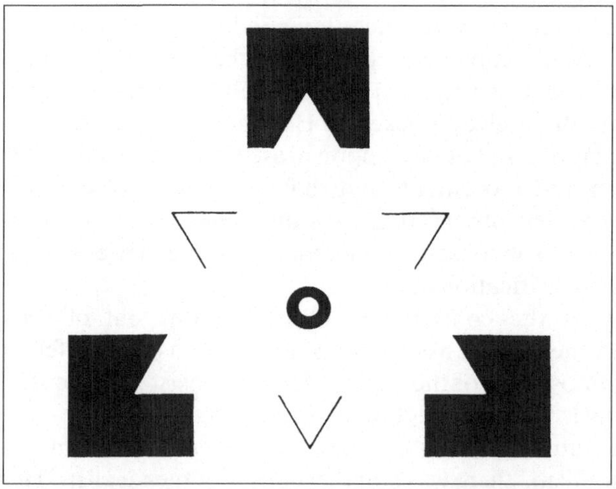

Fig. 11.2. Subjective contours (Kanizsa, 1955). The white triangle (base under) has hardly any objective contours.

showed that the perception of things obeys its own laws, in which the 'sum' of visual elements plays no part. If the curious and clever drawing by Gustave Verbeek (Fig. 11.1) is turned upside down, the picture changes completely, although nothing essential changes in the retinal image. In Figure 11.2 one sees a white triangle, although its contours on the retina are largely absent.

The Gestalt psychologists also had a holistic view of the processes that are started in the brain when forms are observed. The cerebral processes were 'isomorphic' with the psychic image. Thus, when a dog was seen there was a dog-configuration in the brain, undoubtedly distorted, but topologically intact. With foresight, this dog-process was not placed in an atomistic, Newtonian context, but in a 'field.' Thus the retinal images of a large and a small dog could, in the (supposedly electric) field of the brain, give rise to an almost identical tension pattern, a concept that would explain the phenomenon of the constancy of visual objects.

The important discoveries made in neurophysiology, especially in the second half of the nineteenth century, sounded the knell of the above mythology. The pendulum swung back to the elements, thus from holism to reductionism. The findings have already been discussed in the previous chapters: cellular detectors of orientation, contours, disparity and movement. It was soon assumed that, with the right experiments, enough information would be obtained on the cellular level to explain the process of vision. At last the cell would be found in the cat, which could only be stimulated by a mouse, and the motor pathway from that cell to the claw would be traced.

Neurophysiological research has certainly advanced a long way in that direction. In apes, for instance, cells have been found that can only be stimulated by a face. But in spite of all this, vision has not become less of an enigma. It has not been explained how the recognition of a face takes place. That is an almost unanswerable question for a neurophysiologist. The procedure the brain follows to make the activity of many thousands of cells converge to one 'face-cell,' is beyond the reach of experiments. For this reason, in the dialectical development of thought, a new path to the 'whole' is being sought.

The new path leads to the science of information processing. It has become clear that knowledge of individual cells and their receptive fields is inadequate for the understanding of the collective action of thousands of nerve cells. Knowledge of a feather doesn't teach one how a bird flies! It is necessary to make an analysis of the flight system, possibly using a 'computer simulation.' This has also been tried for the analysis of the visual system. When it had been demonstrated that an artificial brain could be the equal of a master chess player, it looked as though it would be easy to make a computer program to distinguish optically between a table and a chair. But nothing could be less true. Vision, which seems to us so simple, was found to be extremely refractory to artificial intelligence. This made people reconsider carefully just how objects are seen. Three steps can be distinguished in this analysis. In the first place, it must be discovered what the essential information in a scene is, which must be selected and made explicit, while details are temporarily ignored. The fundamental question is 'what' exactly must be selected, and for what purpose. After that, the question 'how' follows, the question of the possible procedure. The final question is 'with what': whether our neural apparatus possesses the right machinery to carry out the proposed calculation.

The information theorist finds himself in the no-man's land between the 'input' and the 'output' of vision, but is not entirely alone there. In various ways he can seek confirmation of whether he is on the right path. That may be carefully constructed psychological tests, neurophysiological experiments or neuropathological observations. This field has become 'almost a new intellectual landscape.' The quotation is from David Marr (1945–1980), who was a pioneer in the field of the processing of visual information[1]. He distinguishes three steps in vision: a first sketch of lines and contours, then the perception of surfaces and depth, and finally the construction of three-dimensional images.

CONTOURS, CONTRASTS AND THE PRIMARY SKETCH

In 1865 Ernst Mach (1836–1916), physicist, philosopher, scientific historian and psychologist, saw a curious phenomenon that has been named 'Mach's bands' after him[2] (Fig. 11.3). The figure consists of a series of stripes of uniform, but increasing, brightness placed one beside the other. At each boundary between a darker and a lighter stripe, there is a narrow band of apparently greater brightness on the dark side and an extra dark band on the lighter side. Mach assumed that the bands were due to horizontal connections between the retinal elements. Through these connections a stimulated retinal element could tone down the surrounding elements. In five articles he propounded a mathematical formula for the total of the opposing influences of inhibition and stimulation.

Figure 11.4 gives a diagram of the objective light distribution of the stripes, with below the subjective brightness of the bands. It seems probable that the latter curve is a representation of the neural activity. The diagram shows that, at a boundary between light and dark, the dark is extra dark and the light is extra light. In Chapter 6 we already saw how a ganglion cell has an antagonistically organized receptive field. If light shines on the centre of the field, the cell can be stimulated, while illumination of the periphery has an inhibiting action on the cell's activity. The antagonistic effect can also be the other way round: central inhibition, peripheral stimulation. Cortical cells also have this antagonistic organization. If the whole receptive field of such cells is illuminated, there is no electrical response. This makes these antagonistically organized cells pre-eminently suited to be 'edge detectors,'

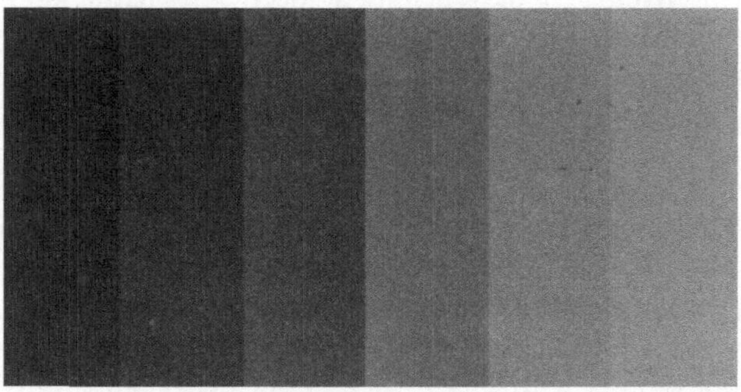

Fig. 11.3. Mach's bands (1865). In this series of uniformly grey stripes becoming steadily darker, each stripe appears to have a light band at the boundary with a darker stripe and a dark band at the boundary with a lighter stripe.

---

[1] Marr, 1982.
[2] Ratliff, 1965.

which register transitions in brightness. The result is a sketch! Even a computer with an 'edge-detecting' program can make such a sketch of an object, as evidenced by Figure 11.5.

It is probable that, when building up perception, the visual system begins with a rough sketch, just like an artist. A sketch has various advantages: it doesn't take much time and makes the essential structures of the subject clear without paying attention to gradations of brightness and details of surfaces. In addition, some cells are responsible for the rough draft, while others have the task of filling in the details. In technical terminology: cells differ in sensitivity to different spatial frequencies.

The edge detectors perform what Descartes (p. 138) had predicted: they produce facts whose 'perfection is often dependent on the degree to which they do not so strongly resemble the things as they might.' Mach also arrives at a similar wording: 'One might say that the retina works schematically and in caricatures. The teleological significance of the process is clear. It is an analogy of abstraction and concept formation.'

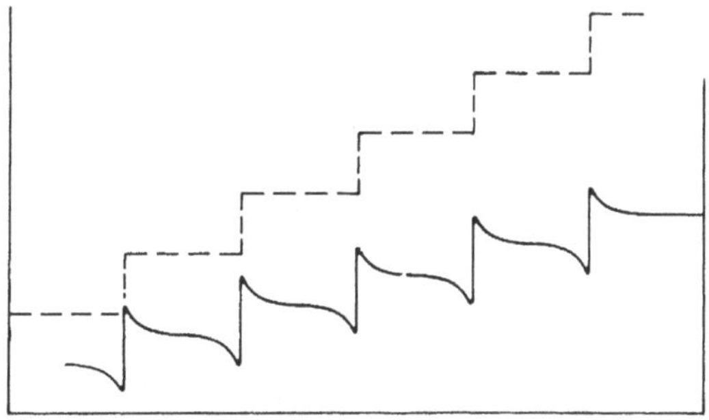

Fig. 11.4. Graph of Mach's bands (dotted line). Horizontally from left to right there are stripes of gradually increasing light reflection. The lower curve (solid line) shows the course of the brightness sensation and the probable neural activity (Cornsweet, 1970).

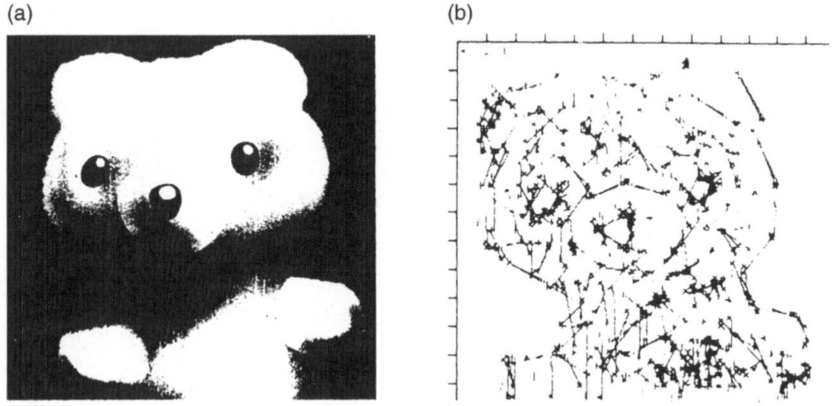

Fig. 11.5. Grey tones and a sketch. The sketch is made by a computer (Frisby, 1979).

As we shall see in the next section, the purpose of the process can be given in a little more detail: the sketch is the first essential for the completion of the surfaces with respect to brightness, colour and depth.

THE PERCEPTION OF SURFACES[3]

This section begins, like the last, with a remarkable illusion. Figure 11.6 shows two discs, half black and half white. A pattern has been made in the dividing line on the left disc, marking the transition—from the outside to the inside—between light and dark, a pattern that must, according to Figure 11.4, make optimal edge detection possible. On the right disc the black section occupies 180 degrees at the periphery, but at the centre the angle is greater. When the discs spin so quickly that no movement can be seen, one would expect that a circular boundary would be seen on the left disc, and that on the right disc the centre would be a little darker than the periphery. But that is not the case: both discs, and not only the right one, have a dark centre! Apparently it is unimportant for the definitive subjective impression whether the whole centre reflects less light or not. In the left disc it is apparently

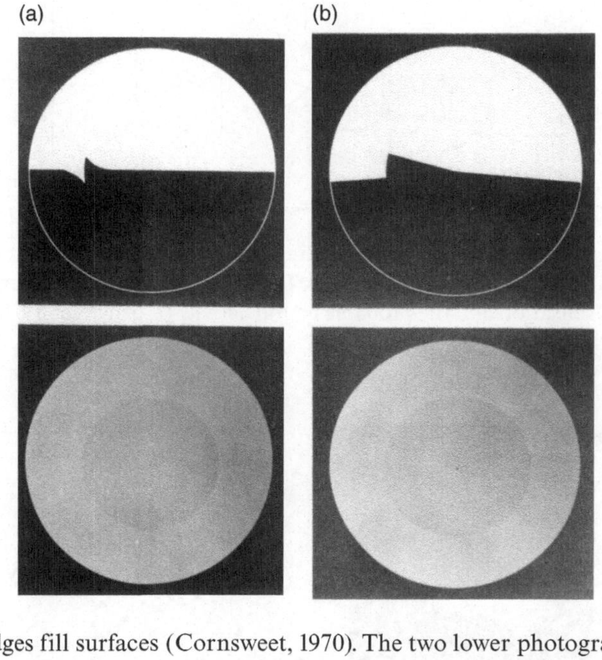

Fig. 11.6. Edges fill surfaces (Cornsweet, 1970). The two lower photographs were made while the discs shown above were spinning. They seem to be almost identical, although in the left photograph the centre reflects as much light as the periphery and that is not the case in the right photograph.

[3] Cornsweet, 1970.

the configuration of the boundary that causes the whole central area to be 'filled in.' The situation is shown in a diagram in Figure 11.7. A shows the objective distribution of light on the revolving discs, B the subjective impression, with Mach bands and filling-in of the centre from the edge inwards. While the objective distribution of light on the discs is different, the subjective impression of the two is the same.

It seems incredible that surfaces can be filled in from the edges, but it has been demonstrated impressively by experiments with images stabilised on the retina. Figure 11.8 shows an apparatus constructed by the Russian biophysicist Yarbus. It is a cap attached by suction to the eye, on which a strong lens is mounted and a holder for a piece of microfilm. When light is shone on the latter it is represented 'stabilised,' completely immobile, on the retina, in spite of the fixational instability of the eye (Fig. 6.12). We shall presume that the microfilm shows an illuminated disc

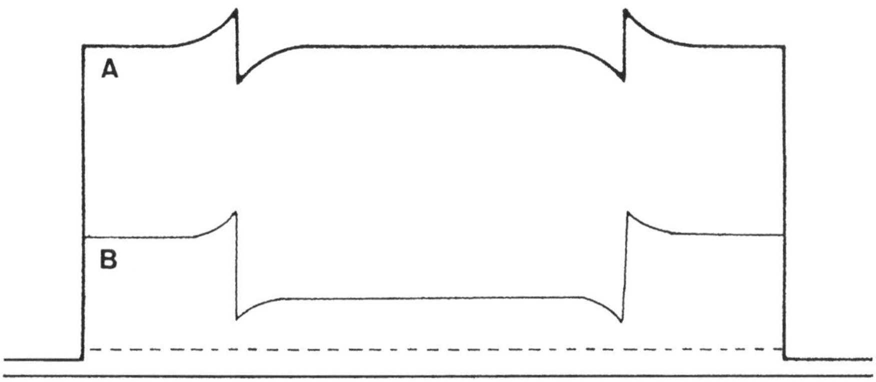

Fig. 11.7. Diagram of Cornsweet's illusion. (A) Objective reflection; (B) 'filling-in' of the central area from the edges.

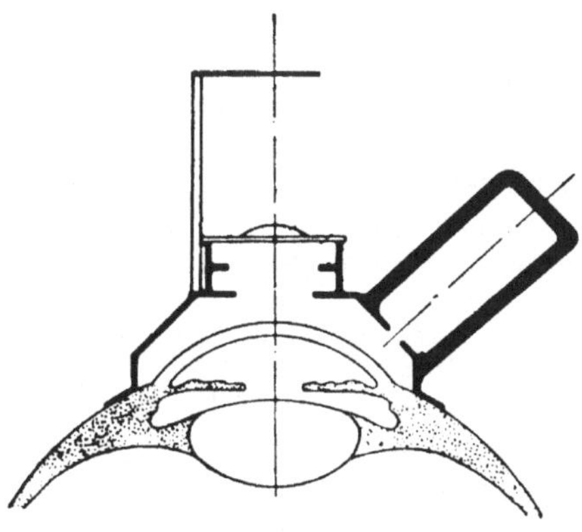

Fig. 11.8. Image stabilisation. A magnifying glass and a micro-film are attached to a contact lens which is fastened by suction to the cornea. The image from the film remains stationary on the retina although the eye is moving. In these circumstances the image is only momentarily visible (Yarbus, 1967).

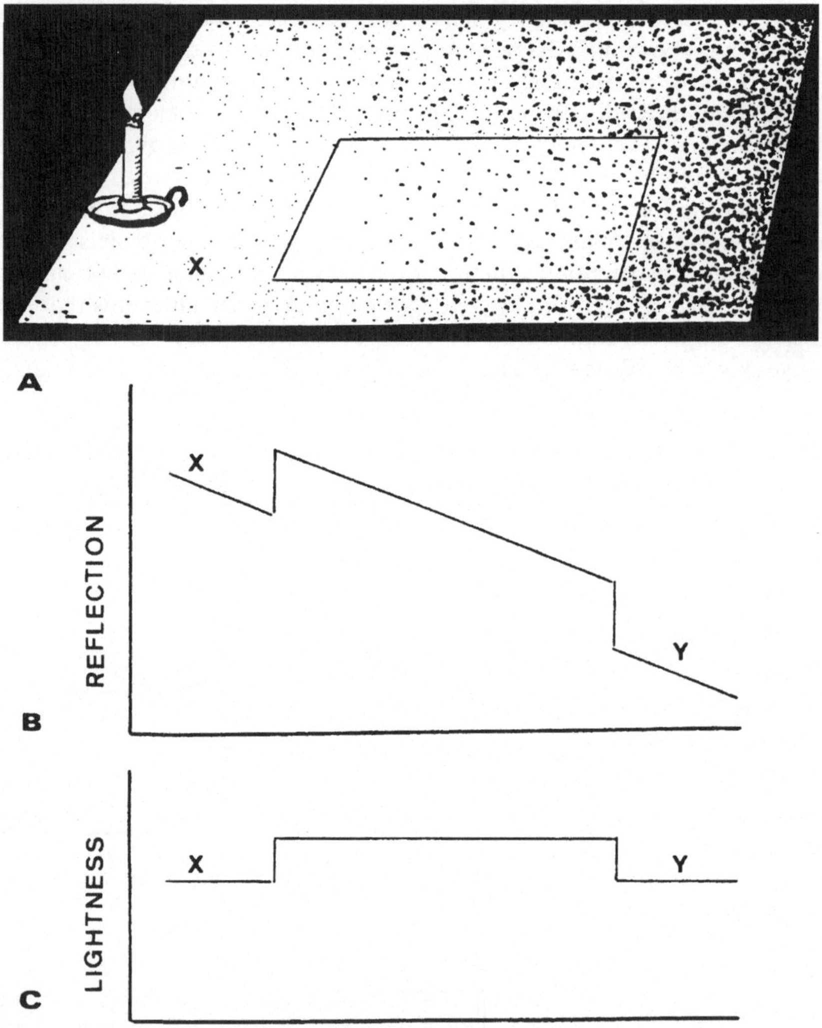

Fig. 11.9. An unevenly illuminated sheet of white paper. (A) White paper on grey table with candle; (B) light reflection along the line X–Y; (C) recognizable uniform white surface, produced by contour detection and reconstruction, as shown in Fig. 11.7 (Crone, 1999).

on a black background. One half of the disc is bright red, the other half bright green. If this picture is shown to someone, an extraordinary thing happens. When the light goes on, he at first sees the disc as it is, but that only lasts a few seconds. Almost immediately the colours become grey and the contours also disappear, so that one uniform grey field is seen. It thus becomes clear that the micro-movements of the eye are essential for vision. Apparently surfaces can only be seen if boundary detectors are continually passing over the transitions of brightness and colour.

We must ask ourselves what purpose is served by this strange operation. Why is the natural contrast (as in the right disc in Fig. 11.6) first eliminated and then replaced by an artificial contrast, generated by a boundary? The answer is: because the visual system is often unable to make much of the first interpretation of the image with its natural contrasts. That can be seen in Figure 11.9A. A candle illuminates a white paper on a grey background. The right side of the white paper is darker than the grey background on the left, close to the candle (Fig. 11.9B). It is clear that this makes it very difficult to interpret the piece of paper as one white surface. In reality, intermediate links are introduced into the recognition process. The sketch is first made, with the help of edge detectors which are only sensitive to sudden changes and not to gradual transitions. Then the lightness of the paper is assessed, as shown in Figure 11.9C.

The experiment with the stabilised retinal image teaches us that it is not only the contours and the brightness which are kept active by moving edges, but also the colour. As colour is not, like brightness, dependent on one variable but on three, the assessment of lightness must be carried out for three independent variables. The benefit of such an assessment is clear: identification of a coloured surface in spite of irregularly coloured light. Such a situation often occurs; for instance, a surface illuminated by a yellow sun, while the shadows reflect the blue sky.

The perception of surfaces from their edges, therefore, makes their recognition easier if they are irregularly illuminated and coloured, but also has a purpose if there are no irregularities. The number of fibres in the optic nerves is limited, compared with the enormous number of image points that make up an image. It would be damaging to the economy of vision if the image points of a uniform surface were to tax the visual information process as greatly as the image points of contours.

12. Seeing Objects in Depth

PERSPECTIVE[1]

Stereoscopic vision, as one of the fundamental elements of spatial vision, was considered in Chapter 7. It is amazingly precise and plays an important part in the identification of near objects. But there are many other factors which enable us to see depth, even in the distance. We shall begin with perspective.

In objective space every object has its position relative to other objects. This relative localisation signifies that no objects are far away and no objects are close by, because there is no observer in relation to whom a distance could be measured; objects have their position in a Cartesian co-ordinate system, the origin of which may be anywhere. Neither can one object cause another object to disappear by overlapping it, because there is no observer in relation to whom an object can be overlapped. A blind man walking in a wood, with only his sense of touch—according to Buffon his *sens géométrique*—available finds himself in the same situation. In visual space the situation is different: the position of the trees is related to the visual egocentre of the observer. Some trees are far away, others nearby, and others are invisible because another tree stands in front of them.

In the chapter on the perception of direction we encountered the two polar co-ordinates of directional vision, but the (monocular) depth co-ordinate was not mentioned. What, in monocular vision, the depth criterion is, is difficult to say. Yet it is abundantly clear that the world we see is filled with distances and depth, even when we close one eye. People have tried to deny this. A famous declaration was made by Bishop Berkeley at the beginning of his *New Theory of Vision* (1709): '*It is, I think, agreed by all that Distance, of itself and immediately, cannot be seen. For, distance being a line directed endwise to the eye, it projects only one point in the fund of the eye, which point remains invariably the same, whether the distance be longer or shorter.*' Here Berkeley makes two obvious mistakes: he makes an unjustifiable leap from psychology to physiology (the flat retinal image) and, in addition, he assumes that the surrounding world contains nothing more than points projected onto the retina instead of material objects. It is precisely the objects which make it possible to see distances. We observe that two men are seen at totally different angles and conclude that the apparently large man is close by and the other at a distance.

---

[1] Edgerton, 1975.

We see that railway tracks, which we know are everywhere at the same distance from each other, appear to meet each other a few miles away (Fig. 12.1).

We call this perspective. And perspective is the basis of monocular depth perception. It can be studied as a branch of projective geometry but, without knowledge of geometry, everyone is familiar with the phenomenon of perspective. Euclid, in his optics, was the first to study the geometry of the visual world. He thought that straight visual rays left the eye and fell onto objects. Objects that no rays fell onto were invisible. The rays were contained in the visual cone. Objects seen at a greater angle appeared to be larger.

Perspective has often been called a 'pictorial' criterion of monocular depth perception. The term can be defended historically, if one takes into consideration that painters, Egyptian, Indian or Chinese, have seldom been much interested in the suggestion of depth. It was only in the Florentine paintings in the Renaissance that 'linear perspective' blossomed. It was discovered by Filippo Brunelleschi, the great architect of the dome of the cathedral in Florence. That was certainly not by chance. It is the geometrical relationships of buildings, in particular, which form a challenge for a naturalistic representation of depth. And pictures had to be naturalistic! Ideally, a picture had to look as if one was looking through the frame at

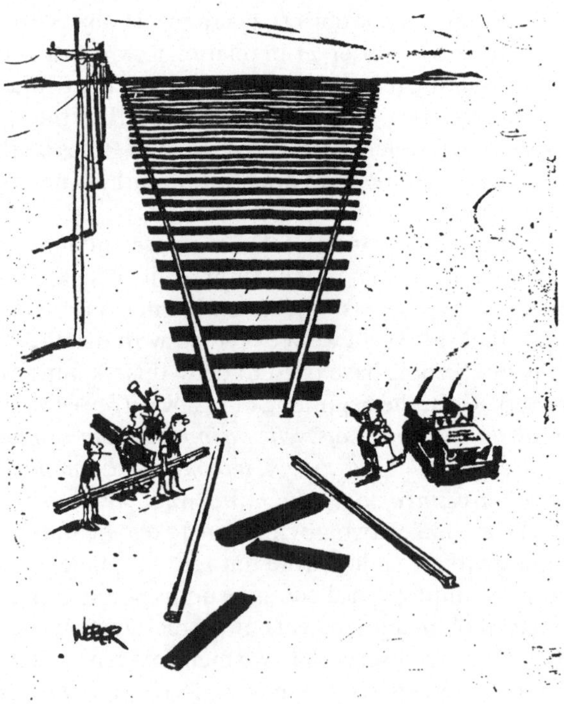

Fig. 12.1. Perspective gone haywire. 'Look here, you men, shouldn't that be the other way round?'

reality. The painting had to be, as it were, a section through the Euclidean cone, which has its apex in the eye and its base on the object. Brunelleschi tried to reproduce this situation by an ingenious method. In order to draw the Florentine Baptisterium he bored a hole in a panel, stood with his back to the Baptisterium and looked through the hole at a mirror, which projected the building onto the artist's panel. He drew a theoretical line on the panel, representing the horizon at eye-level, and discovered that the parallel lines of the building converged to 'disappearing points' on the horizon.

The theory of perspective was given by the humanist Alberti (Fig. 12.2). It is an application of Euclid's optical thesis that measurements are seen at a smaller angle the further away they are. As an aid to drawing in perspective, Alberti used a veil, divided into squares by thick threads, stretched between his eye and the object. In this way he saw the proportions of the object in the way that they had to be drawn on a flat surface. Later artists used the *camera obscura*, although they did not know that the apparatus resembled the human eye to an amazing degree. The principle of the camera obscura had been known for a long time, but the first picture of one dates from 1544 (Fig. 12.3). It is a real room with an opening, and opposite the opening a white screen on which the inverted image of the outside world is visible.

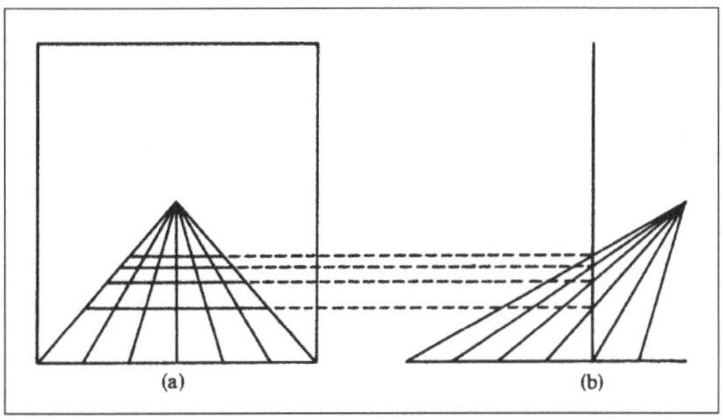

Fig. 12.2. Alberti's perspective construction (1435). Parallel lines perpendicular to the surface of the drawing converge to a disappearing point (a). Evenly spaced lines parallel to the surface of the drawing come to lie, according to (b), steadily closer to each other in the direction of the disappearing point (after Lindberg, 1976).

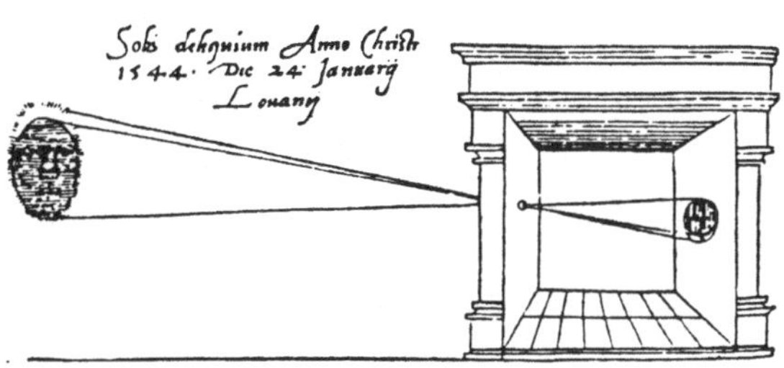

Fig. 12.3. The oldest picture of a camera obscura. The 1544 eclipse of the sun is shown upside down (after Hammond, 1981).

Perspective ruled painting until the second half of the nineteenth century. Then the camera arrived. This excellent copy of the human eye produced pictures with faultless perspective. Too faultless, as many a tourist discovered when he directed his camera upwards to get the whole of a building into the picture. Then convergence of the vertical lines occurred, which was aesthetically undesirable and in disagreement with our feeling that gravity demands parallel vertical constructions. After the invention of photography, pictorial artists lost their interest in perspective. Picasso painted faces in profile, in which the hidden eye moved onto the visible side of the face, just as, in evolution, the lower eye of flat-fish moved to the upper side.

OTHER PICTORIAL DEPTH EFFECTS

Atmospheric perspective was also described by Alberti. Distant views often have a different (bluer) colour than near ones.

Shadow was eliminated from the first recognition of a surface as a surface (Fig. 11.9). At a later stage in surface identification, the brightness gradient is important for the estimation of depth in the surface. Figure 12.4 is nothing more than a circle; when it is shaded it becomes a ball. It is interesting to see the inversion of the depth effect with certain sorts of shading. It is one of the experiences of everyday life that light comes from above. Convex vertical structures are therefore usually light at the top and dark at the bottom. If Figure 12.4 is turned upside down, one's first thought is not that light is coming from below but that one is looking into a hollow.

Overlapping is perhaps the weightiest criterion for depth. When one person on a group photograph is largely overlapped by another, it is certain that the latter is in front of the former.

NECKER'S CUBE

Figure 12.5a shows the famous cube drawn in 1832 by the Swiss naturalist Necker. The cube demonstrates what happens when four criteria for the estimation of depth are absent: stereoscopy, perspective, shadow and overlapping. We know that the drawing represents a spatial figure, but the cube has no clear front or back. That produces a peculiar sensation: if you look at the cube for some time the front and the back continually change places. This illusion can be suppressed by perspective, shading, and especially by letting the back be overlapped by the front (Fig. 12.5b).

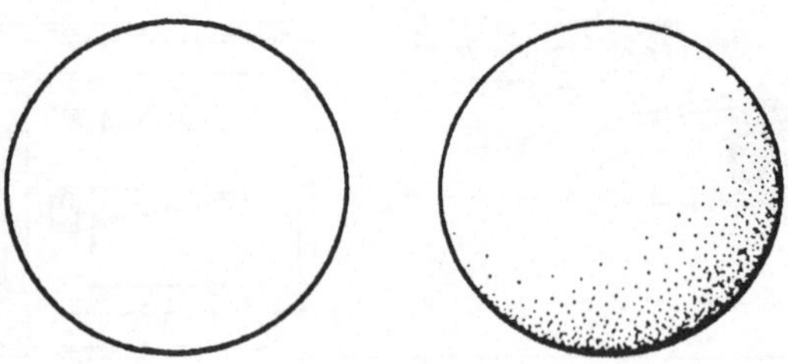

Fig. 12.4. Depth through shadow. The right figure seems to be a ball, but when it is held upside down, it looks like a hollow.

The angle at which one looks at a (real) cube makes a lot of difference. If one looks with one eye from some distance at the centre of the front, one sees only a square and no cube. When a corner of the front coincides with the corresponding corner of the back, it is also difficult to recognize a cube: a two-dimensional regular hexagon is more likely (Fig. 12.6). One only needs to turn the cube a very little to make it directly recognizable. With this observation we arrive at a new aspect of depth perception: depth perception through movement. This must now occupy our attention.

DEPTH PERCEPTION THROUGH MOVEMENT

Perspective vision is an important means of seeing monocular depth, but it is not the only one. The hole in Brunelleschi's panel discloses the origin of perspective, but also its limitation: perspective vision is a static occupation. In normal life we move about in the space around us and find many indications of depth in *movement parallax*. Someone driving past a double row of trees, sees the front row move backwards relative to the back row. A pilot also orientates himself on the basis of

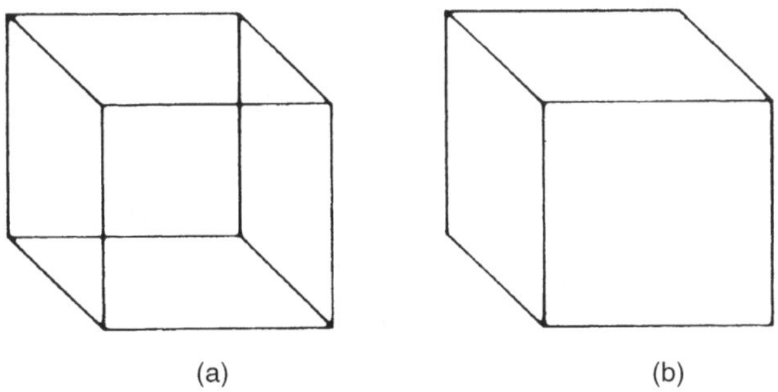

Fig. 12.5. Necker's cube. In cube (a) front and back alternate continually. When (b) opaque surfaces cover the ribs at the back, the alternation takes place much less frequently.

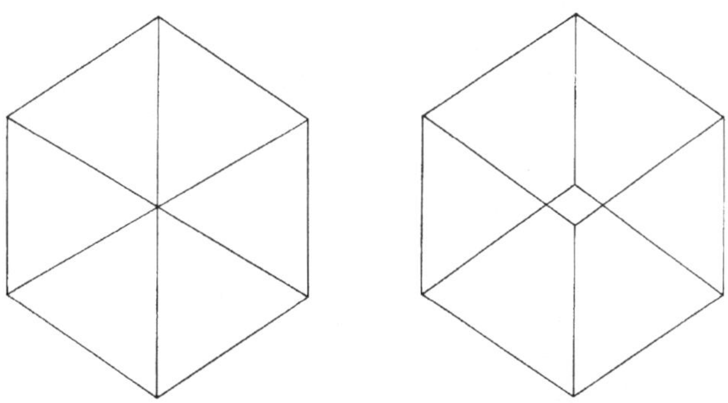

Fig. 12.6. The left figure is a regular hexagon, in which a cube can be recognized with difficulty. A small change in position of the cube (right) makes it easy to recognize.

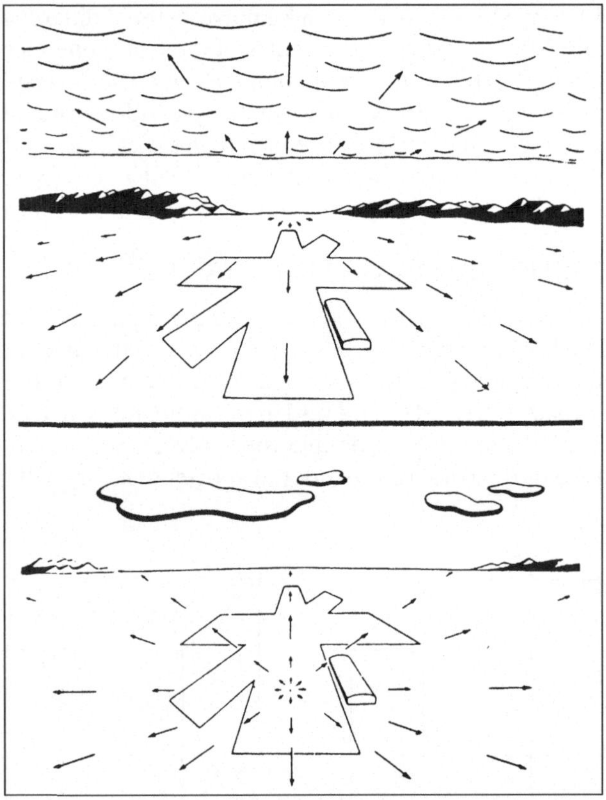

Fig. 12.7. Depth localisation by receding contours (Gibson, 1950). Above: when a pilot is flying straight ahead; below: when he is starting to land.

receding contours (Fig. 12.7). But we are not dependent on motor traffic for the estimation of depth. Even moving the head from side to side is an important aid to depth perception. When we move our heads sideways, things alter their position more the nearer they are; the relative position of distant objects does not change. A head movement need not be large—for instance, only 10 cm—to provide important information about depth. For people with normal sight, smaller movements have no purpose: stereoscopy then takes over depth perception.

THE OBJECTIVE FORM OF OBJECTS[2]

The identification of contours, surfaces, depth and measurements has led to a three-dimensional analysis, but it is a specification that is strictly coupled with the observer's perspective. Objects are seen from an, essentially random, visual angle. For the recognition of objects that is a disadvantage. It would be better if the objects

[2] Marr, 1982.

could be removed from the individual visual space and reduced to a more objective spatial form. A three-dimensional model like that would be more suitable for comparison with a model stored in the memory.

What is 'a more objective spatial form?' This question can be answered quite easily. The vertical is an undisputed spatial co-ordinate, determined by gravity. If one adds two horizontal co-ordinates, perpendicular to each other, one has Descartes' system. This is an excellent system for an architect, but a choreographer can also use it to pinpoint the position of a dancer on the stage.

The Cartesian system is unsuitable for a woodworker or handicraftsman. He doesn't want to be tied to a vertical co-ordinate or the condition that the axes must be perpendicular to each other. When a gardener is looking for a hoe, it doesn't interest him whether the hoe is lying on the ground or standing straight up or leaning against a wall. A hoe is an object with a long main axis, the handle, onto the end of which a transverse piece of iron is attached which is flattened for a short distance at an angle which is not perpendicular to the first two co-ordinates. Like this—in its own axial system, centred in the object—the hoe is engraved in the gardener's memory, and like this, the visual percept must be presented to the memory in order to be recognized.

The following step in the build-up of the visual world is therefore the construction of the visual objects in their own objective co-ordinate systems. The magic machine which must perform this task is called by Marr the 'image-space converter.' The technical realisation does not seem to be very difficult. An ingenious machine can undoubtedly be invented that can convert the perspective-stereoscopic image into another system. The brain also has the necessary 'wiring' for this purpose. The sensation of touch (including the muscular sense, etc.) already makes use of an axial system centred in the object for its analysis of form. Therefore, all that the 'image-space converter' has to do, is to perform a transformation from the perspective-visual world to the world of touch.

At this point we cross the threshold of the strictly visual. We find ourselves in an intermediate area in which the spatial systems of two special senses are co-ordinated. It is tempting to include the sense of equilibrium in the discussion at the same time. For that sense the vertical is an inalienable co-ordinate. If the sense of equilibrium also makes its contribution, we probably finally arrive at a Cartesian model of space. The phenomenal space postulated by Kant as the a priori form of perception, is then not far away (although that sort of space cannot serve as a standard for geometry and physics).

The action of the 'image-space converter' can be described in detail. It is essential that the description begins with the main issue and ends with the details. This is simple for the description of a walking-stick with a handle, for a crumpled newspaper it is almost impossible.

How far one can get with a simple description of main and auxiliary axes can be seen in Figure 12.8, in which Marr shows animals modelled from pipe-cleaners. Recognition of surfaces is not even necessary. A vertebrate land-animal consists of trunk, neck, head, and two or four limbs, in variable proportions and sizes. We can easily look up the visual three-dimensional model in our memory, which contains a catalogue of vertebrates.

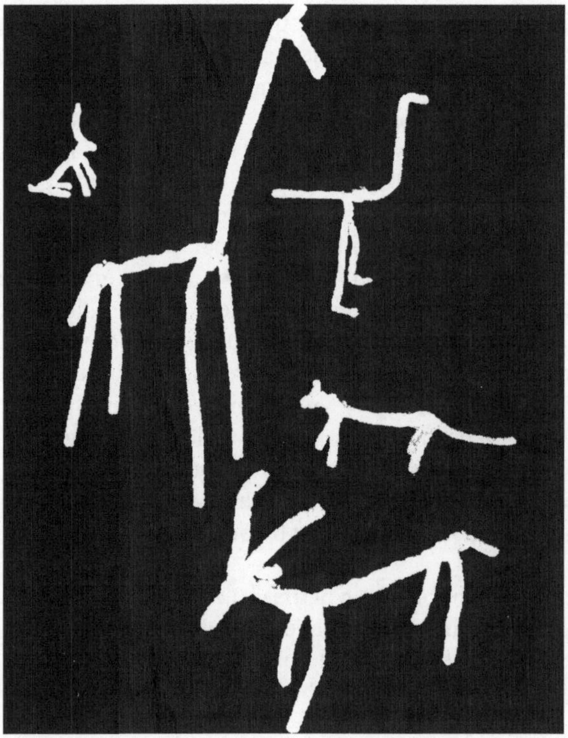

Fig. 12.8. Animals from pipe cleaners (Marr, 1982). The length and position of a small number of axes is enough to make many animals recognizable.

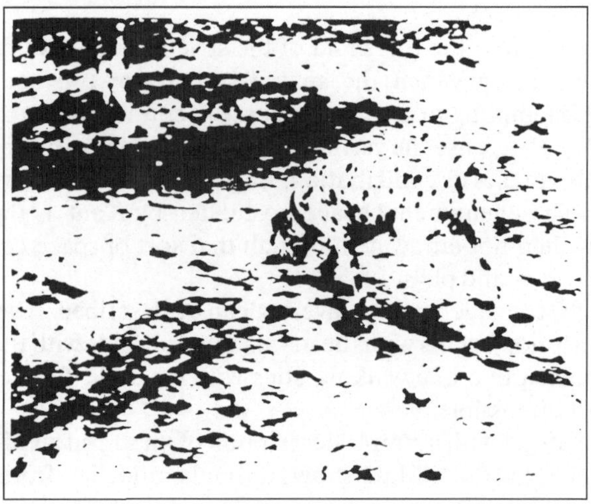

Fig. 12.9. Dalmatian with its nose to the ground. An object can be recognized on the basis of a few features well imprinted in the memory, even without a 'primary sketch,' surface recognition or stereoscopy (after R.C. James).

It is suggested above that the recognition of objects is built up on the lines of an established system. First, a rough sketch of the object is made, then the surfaces are filled with their patterns, depth and colour. After that, the perspective description is objectified and schematised into a three-dimensional model. Finally, the cognitive element comes into play: looking up the percept in memory's catalogue. This progress from sensory to cognitive recognition processes is certainly not the only possibility. Sometimes the memory 'descends' to a visual detail at an early stage in the visual information analysis. Figure 12.9 gives an example. Without the contours of the dog being drawn, let alone a three-dimensional model of the dog being made, memory steps in. On the basis of one small detail, the snout and ear area, it tells us: this is a dog; on account of the spots, it says: it is a Dalmatian! But in many cases recognition occurs in steps. Then perceptual and cognitive contributions combine to produce the definite identification.

This is not the place to expatiate on the neurophysiological aspects of memory. The hippocampus appears to play a very important role in this process, a cortical area lying on the inner and lower side of the temporal lobe. There is undoubtedly a multi-modal representation of space in the hippocampus, in an objectified three-dimensional form.

13. The Perception of Size

INTRODUCTION

The perception of size, an extremely important aspect of the perception of objects, is a branch of the psychology of vision. The physiologist, who begins with the retina and ends with an eye movement or other motor reaction, has nothing to do with it. This is because the retina only registers angular measurements, while the size of a visual object depends on the distance as well as the visual angle. A short distance can be estimated with the help of stereoscopy, but at greater distances the stationary eye is not able to estimate independently the distance and the visual angle by physiological means. This can be easily demonstrated by an experiment. In a completely dark passage a 30-cm band of light at 3 metres cannot be distinguished from a 3-metre band of light at 30 metres.

Nevertheless, much has been written about 'size constancy,' the fact that size perception is independent of distance. Size constancy is based on knowledge, not on physiology. At whatever distance and visual angle something is seen, a bicycle is in our experience always equally large, and is seen as equally large at all distances. The same is true for people, the steps of a staircase, and all other objects which we know do not vary much in size.

Of course there is an intermediate area: there are large and small trees, large and small statues. The key to the correct assessment of size is perspective. In surroundings with suggestive perspective one knows that objects are seen under a smaller visual angle as they get further away—and vice versa—and estimates the size of the object by its position in the perspective. Many optical illusions are based on severing the relation between perspective depth and angular size. A typical example is the corridor illusion (Fig. 13.1).

EMMERT'S LAW[1]

Emmert, a German scholar who was interested in the physiology and psychology of vision, wrote an article in 1881 on the size of after-images. After-images (which can easily be produced by looking at a photographic flash from nearby) have a certain size on the retina which does not change, but their *apparent* size is dependent on the

[1] Emmert, 1881; ten Doesschate, 1930.

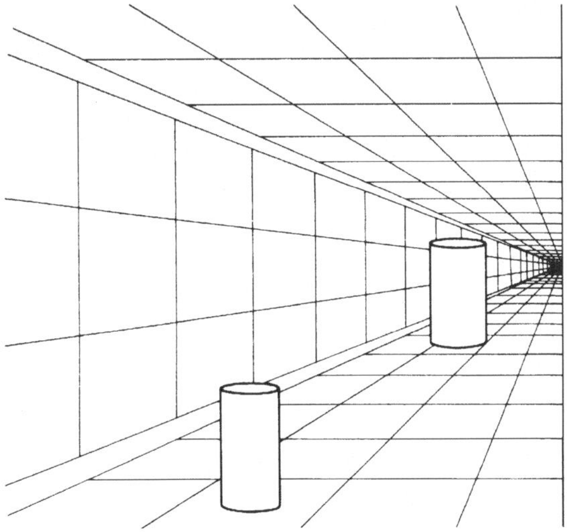

Fig. 13.1. The corridor illusion.

distance from which one looks. If someone sees an after-image on a book lying open in front of him, the after-image is small, but if he is looking at the wall it is large. The tendency to localise the after-image on the surface that one is looking at, is an example of the *horror profundi* that we encountered when considering 'random dot patterns' and the 'two-nail illusion.' Vision refuses depth where it is not necessary.

But there is more in Emmert's law that reminds us of stereoscopic vision: at the limit of stereoscopic vision, Emmert's law (the linear relationship between the apparent size of the after-image and the distance at which it is seen) loses its validity. After about 50 m, the limit of useful stereoscopic vision, an after-image ceases to grow. If one 'projects' an after-image onto the blue sky, thus very far away, its apparent size is not larger than when one projects the image onto a wall at a distance of 20 or 30 metres. This provides us with the key to an ancient puzzle, which will be expounded in the next section.

THE SIZES OF THE SUN AND THE MOON: A HISTORICAL DIGRESSION[2]

It is well known that the sun and the moon appear larger just above the horizon than at their zenith. This is generally called the 'moon illusion.' Scholars have been racking their brains about this *relative* difference in size for thousands of years, usually without asking themselves what the size of the sun and the moon is that we see. Nevertheless, the problem of the *absolute* phenomenal size of the sun and the moon will have to be solved before we can begin on the moon illusion.

The pre-Socratic philosopher Heraclitus was the first to give an opinion on the size of the sun. A famous quotation from Heraclitus is: *The size of the sun is the same*

[2] Hershenson, 1989; Schönbeck, 1998; Crone, 2000.

as the size of a human foot. Every discussion about the size of our two most important celestial bodies or the moon illusion begins with Heraclitus. But may we expect psychological conceptions from one of the earliest Greek philosophers? Did Heraclitus really think that the apparent size of the sun was the same as that of the human foot, or did he allow himself to be guided by all sorts of mythological arguments? Greek commentators soon decided that Heraclitus was really describing the apparent size of the sun. Incidentally, later investigators came to the same conclusion as Heraclitus. A century ago a German psychologist stated that the sun seems to be as big as a soup-plate. Heraclitus thus estimated the sun, which has a diameter of 30 minutes of arc, to be at a distance of about 40 metres. I shall presently try to explain why that is so.

For thousands of years strong feelings have been aroused by the question why the moon (or the sun) seems larger just above the horizon than high in the sky. Aristotle already posed this question. He thought that it was due to the air perspective, which caused the moon to be less bright on the horizon. Air perspective is an indication of great distance, and thus of increased apparent size. Aristotle knew that the greater apparent size of the moon above the horizon was an optical illusion. He didn't believe that the rising or setting moon was closer to the earth, and for this reason appeared to be larger. He could not believe this because his world consisted of the earth, which was at the centre, surrounded by *concentric* circles of sun, moon and stars. Later Greeks did not deviate from this conception of the world either. The Stoic astronomer Cleomedes wrote: 'when the sun culminates it *appears* to be closest; when it rises or sets it *appears* to be further away.'

Ptolemy described an important observation in his *Optica*: that the objective angular size (which is about 30 minutes of arc for both the sun and the moon) is the same at the horizon and at the zenith. The moon illusion is thus no physico-optical, but a psychological illusion.

About 1000 AD, the great Arabian scholar Ibn-al Haytham (called Alhazen in the West) was in agreement with Ptolemy. He gave two, purely psychological, explanations of the moon illusion. In the first place, it is because the firmament appears to be flattened. In the second place, it is on account of intervening things that the moon at the horizon seems larger than when it is high in the sky.

Let us first consider Alhazen's first explanation (the firmament is an inverted dish, stretching further to the sides than upwards; therefore the low moon is localised further away and thus seen as larger than when it is high in the sky). A flattened firmament was not an original idea of Alhazen's. Empedocles[3], the Sicilian philosopher who was only a few decades younger than Heraclitus, had said something similar. In the best days of Arabian culture, the flattening of the firmament was a familiar idea. One only needs to read a verse of Omar Khayyam to understand this:

> And that inverted bowl we call the sky,
> Whereunder crawling coop't we live and die,
> Lift not thy hands to *it* for help—for it
> Rolls impotently on as thou and I.

---

[3] Bollack, 1965.

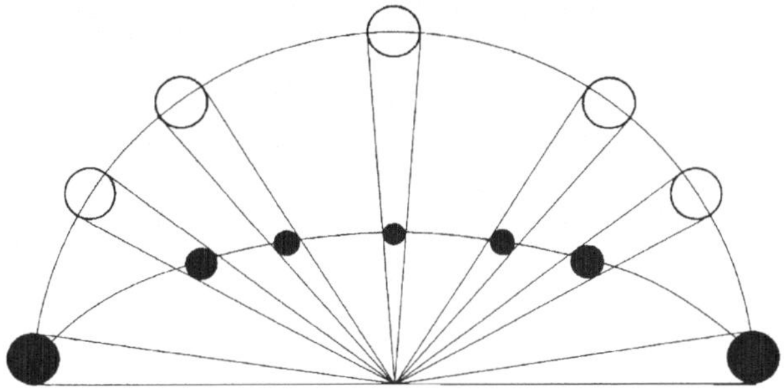

Fig. 13.2. The moon illusion (Smith, 1728). One thinks of the firmament as flattened. The moon, which is always seen at the same angle, appears bigger at the horizon than at its zenith.

Alhazen's first explanation of the moon illusion held its ground for centuries. The astronomer and mathematician Robert Smith published in his *Optics* in 1728 a diagram of the connection between the flattening of the firmament and the moon illusion (Fig. 13.2). Ten Doesschate (1930) investigated the validity of Emmert's law and described how there was a limit to the increase in size of the after-image. He declared that that was the explanation of the flattening of the firmament. If the limitation of Emmert's law is a consequence of the equidistance principle of stereoscopic vision, it is natural that the apparent height of the firmament coincides with the limit of stereoscopic vision, let us say about 50 metres. In this way, Alhazen's first explanation of the moon illusion, the flattened firmament, is reduced to a quality of stereoscopic space.

But Alhazen's second explanation (the influence of intervening things) can also be reduced to modern interpretations of spatial vision. In 1962, the American psychologists Kaufman and Rock measured, with an ingenious apparatus, the apparent difference in the size of artificial moons at their zenith and at the horizon. They demonstrated conclusively that the influence of 'intervening things' was greatest when the intervening things were ordered in a perspective that suggested great depth. The moon illusion is thus based on two characteristics of visual space: the limited range of stereoscopic space and the projective structure of perspective space.

14. The Neurophysiology and Neuropathology of the Perception of Objects[1]

INTRODUCTION

The perception of objects requires global processes in which many elementary occurrences are bundled. Neurophysiology, which has mainly been concentrated on the receptive fields of individual cells, has difficulty in unravelling complicated networks. Nevertheless, neurophysiological discoveries have been made of higher processes of vision taking place beyond the primary visual cortex. As already has been mentioned, in apes cells have been found in the temporal lobe which are particularly sensitive to faces. It is remarkable that some cells only react to a face presented in a certain perspective, while others react irrespective of the position of the face: they are thus sensitive to a face in an objective axial system.

Neurology sees the recognition of objects in a different perspective. Disturbances in object recognition are called *agnosias*. There are many kinds of agnosias, because different cortical areas are equipped for different tasks in the recognition of objects. If a key is only recognized when it has been felt, there is visual agnosia. *Alexia* has been known for more than a century: it is the inability to read, although sight and language comprehension are intact. The cortical lesion that causes alexia is situated in the transitional area between the visual and language areas in the dominant half of the brain. *Prosopagnosia* is a remarkable example of visual agnosia, it is the inability to recognize faces. A child appears to see well, but only recognizes its mother when she begins to speak. In cortical achromatopsia, unilateral or total inability to recognize colours, a special cerebral area is affected (V4).

The distribution of the visual functions over a large number of cortical areas is not devoid of pragmatism. Efficient communication between various parts of the brain which must keep in close contact with each other, is only possible if these parts are situated as close to each other as possible and have the shortest possible connections. It would not be practical if the area for the visual recognition of letters was a long way away from the area for language. Colour information, which is often

[1] Grüsser and Landis, 1991; Zeki, 1993.

not important (for reading and the recognition of movement, for instance), can better be stored separately, so that it can be summoned where necessary. If all visual functions were concentrated in one place, the 'telephone exchange' would be heavily overtaxed.

UNSOLVED PROBLEMS

Knowledge of the dispersion of the numerous functions of the brain just described is nothing new, but does raise the urgent question, how is it possible for us to see in our minds *one* world, in which objects and animals of different colours and shapes move or stand still in different positions, while we at the same time meet people whom we recognize? The brain accommodates the world in many small rooms, but the mind sees the world on one stage.

It is not so easy to position the mental faculty precisely. Soemmering, the famous German anatomist who first described the retinal fovea centralis (as a minute hole in the centre of the retina), published a pamphlet in 1786 with the name: *Über das Organ der Seele* (On the Organ of the Soul). He placed the seat of the soul, following in Galen's footsteps, in the fluid in the ventricles of the brain. He dedicated his pamphlet to a man whom he greatly admired, Immanuel Kant. Kant, who called himself the dissector of the invisible man, wrote a friendly thank-you note to the dissector of the visible man. He also added an extensive exposition on the seat of the soul. His first objection was that such an unstructured mass as water could not possibly be the seat of the immensely complicated structure of the human psyche. His second objection was more basic: we can say that the individual mind is attached to a physical individual, but its position cannot be more precisely specified. Where is the pain caused by a corn on my toe? Its position cannot be determined by physical means. And where in my mental world do I see the red rose planted at the back of the garden by the gardener?

This is the crucial problem in the science of the special senses, which is a synthesis of psychology, concerned with the phenomenal, and physiology, which has just thrown the phenomenal overboard.

Galileo wrote, in his *Saggiatore* (1623), a famous declaration of the principles of natural science. I quote two passages:

> Philosophy is written in this grand book, the Universe, which stands continually open to our gaze. But the book cannot be understood unless one first learns to comprehend the language and read the letters in which it is composed. It is written in the language of mathematics, and its characters are triangles, circles and other geometrical figures without which it is humanly impossible to understand a single word of it; without these, one wanders about in a dark labyrinth. (. . .) To excite in us tastes, colours and sounds, I believe that nothing is in us except shapes, numbers and slow and rapid movements. I think that if ears, tongues and noses were removed, shapes, numbers and motions would remain, but not odours, tastes or sounds. The latter, I believe, are nothing more than names, when separated from living beings.

Galileo (1564–1642) says implicitly here that all knowledge of the Universe can be reduced to knowledge of material things. (It should surprise no-one that Galileo had problems with the church; but that the Vatican has recently apologised for its attitude towards him is more surprising.) Even in the third millennium Galileo has orthodox followers, renowned scholars, some awarded the Nobel Prize, who are convinced that everything mental can be reduced to material processes.

But the psychologists too, who are convinced of the irreducibility of the mental, phenomenal world, can invoke one of the great thinkers of the past. Gottfried Wilhelm Leibnitz (1646–1716) wrote:

> It must be confessed, moreover, that perception and that which depends on it are inexplicable by mechanical causes, that is, by figures and motions. And, supposing that there were a machine so constructed as to think, feel and have perception, we could conceive of it as enlarged and yet preserving the same proportions, so that we might enter it as into a mill. And this granted, we should only find on visiting it, pieces which push one against the other, but never anything by which to explain a perception, and that which depends on it.

Workers in the natural sciences need not lie awake at night wrestling with the problem of whether the mental can be 'reduced' to the material. The theoretical natural sciences can easily do without the sensory qualities. But students of the sensory sciences cannot escape questions about the relationship of the two disciplines.

Sensory science is a *mésalliance* of psychology and natural science. Between the two there is an *incompatibilité d'humeurs*. Their first child was a dwarf, which was therefore called *homunculus*, a little man that was so small (much smaller than the homunculus in Goethe's Faust) that it could penetrate into the substance of the brain. He did not need Leibnitz' large mill. He looked round in the brain (where everything was upside down) and translated what he found into the language of the phenomenal world, in short, he turned the world back the right way up. The homunculus was, and still is, laughed at by the practitioners of natural science, but he got a large number of little brothers and sisters who did the same work (called Copulus 1, Copula 2, etc.), and have been able to survive up to the present day. One returned from a visit to V4 and said that he had seen 'blue.' Another arrived at an area in the temporal lobe and reported that he had been stared at by all sorts of faces. The findings of all these *Copuli* (we call them 'coupling hypotheses'—linking propositions—now) aroused the suspicion that both Galileo and Leibnitz were wrong, although nobody could understand what the real explanation was.

We still cannot understand it at all. Will Copulus 257 ever report that he has found where Free Will is situated? Will Copula 4324, after a journey through a tangle of neurons and synapses, return into the phenomenal world with Chopin's *Nocturnes*? It all sounds ridiculous. Thoughts like these must be based on a simple philosophical error, a category mistake, like that sketched on p. 17.

Dubois-Reymond, the father of electrophysiology, delivered a speech in 1872 on the limits of natural science. He declared that one should not search too far, and need not ask questions about morals and art. He made a distinction between the things that we don't know yet (*ignoramus*) and the things that we shall never know. About this *ignorabimus* he made the following interesting remark: 'It is the problem of sensory sensation, not the problem of Free Will, that lies beyond the realm of analytical mechanics.' Even in the study of something so matter-of-fact as vision, we discover that we shall never decipher certain things by pure natural science. As a Dutch proverb says: 'If you hunt with a cat, you only catch mice.' If we try to hunt down the secrets of the visual world with natural science techniques, we shall only find chemical formulas, nerve tracts and electric potentials. That is a great deal, but not enough.

References

Aguilonius, F. (1613): *Opticorum Libri Sex*. Antwerpen.

Alhazen: see Vitello (1270).

Apkarian, P., Bour L.J., Barth, P.G., Wenniger-Prick, L., Verbeeten Jr, B. (1995): Non-decussating retinal-fungal fibre syndrome. An inborn achiasmatic malformation associated with visuotopic misrouting, visual evoked potential, ipsilateral asymmetry and nystagmus. *Brain 118*, 1195–1216.

Ariëns Kappers, C.U. (1917): Verschijnselen van neurobiotaxis in het optische stelsel. *Psychiat. Neurol. Bl. (Amst.) 21*, 320–365.

Ariëns Kappers, C.U. (1927): On neurobiotaxis. A psychical law in the structure of the nervous system. *Acta Psychiat. (Kbh.) 2*, 118–145.

Bannister, R. (1622): *A treatise of 113 Diseases of the Eyes and the Eyelids*. London.

Bargmann, W. (1977): *Histologie und Mikroskopische Anatomie des Menschen*. Georg Thieme Verlag, Leipzig.

Barlow, H.B., Blakemore, C., Pettigrew, J.D. (1967): The neural mechanism of binocular depth discrimination. *J. Physiol. 193*, 327–342.

Bartisch, G. (1583): *Ophthalmodouleia. Das ist Augendienst*. Dresden.

Berkeley, G. (1709): *An Essay towards a New Theory of Vision*. Dublin.

Berkeley, G. (1710): *A Treatise Concerning the Principles of Human Knowledge*. Dublin.

Bidloo, G. (1715): *De Oculis et Visu Variorum Animalium; Observationes Physico-anatomicae*. Leiden.

Birch, E.E., Stager, D. (1985): Monocular acuity and stereopsis in infantile esotropia. *Invest. Ophthalmol. Vis. Sci. 26*, 1624.

Bishop, P.O. (1975): Binocular Vision. In: *Adler's Physiology of the Eye*. Mosby Comp, St. Louis.

Bollack, J. (1965): Empédocle. TI: *Introduction á l'Ancienne Physique*. Les Éditions de Minuit, Paris.

Brazier, M.A.B. (1984): *A History of Neurophysiology in the 17th and 18th Centuries*. Raven Press, New York.

Campbell, F.W., Gubitsch, R.W. (1966): Optical quality of the human eye. *J. Physiol. 186*, 558.

Campbell, F.W., Robson, J.G. (1969): Application of Fourier analysis to the visibility of gratings. *J. Physiol. 197*, 551–566.

Charpentier, A. (1886): Sur une illusion visuelle. *C.R. Acad. Sci. 102*, 1155–1157.

Cheselden, W. (1728): An Account of some Observations made by a young Gentleman, who was born blind, or lost his Sight so early, that he had no Remembrance of ever having seen, and wa couch'd between 13 and 14 Years of Age. *Phil. T. Roy. Soc. 402*, 447–450.

Cogan, D.G. (1948): *Neurology of the Ocular Muscles*. Charles C. Thomas, Springfield, Ill.

Copernicus, N. (1543): *De Revolutionibus Orbium Coelestium Libri Sex*. Nürnberg.

Cornsweet, T. (1970): *Visual Perception*. Academic Press, New York and London.
Crone, R.A., Velzeboer C.M.J. (1956): Statistics on strabismus in the Amsterdam youth. Researches into the origin of strabismus. *Arch. Ophthalmol. 55*, 455–470.
Crone, R.A. (1964): *Scheelzien*. Swets & Zeitlinger, Amsterdam.
Crone, R.A. (1969): Heterophoria. *Albrecht von Graefes Arch. Klin. Exp. Ophthalmol. 177*, 52–74.
Crone, R.A., Verduyn Lunel, H.F.E. (1969): Autokinesis and the perception of movement: the physiology of eccentric fixation. *Vision Res. 9*, 89–101.
Crone, R.A., Leuridan, O.M.A. (1973): Tolerance for Aniseikonia. *Albrecht von Graefes Arch. Klin. Exp. Ophthalmol. 188*, 1–22.
Crone, R.A. (1973): *Diplopia*. American Elsevier Company, Inc., New York. Reprint (1993); C.E.R.E.S. Cercle d'Études de la Strabologie, Éditions et Materiels Scientifiques, Paris.
Crone, R.A. (1977a): Amblyopia: The pathology of motor disorders in amblyopic eyes. *Doc. Ophthalmol. Proc. Ser. 11*, 9–18.
Crone, R.A. (1977b): Die Physiologie der Netzhautperipherie. *Ber. Deut. Ophthalmol. Ges. 74*, 17–21.
Crone, R.A., Sanjoto Hardjowijoto (1979): What is normal binocular vision? *Doc. Ophthalmol. 47*, 163–199.
Crone, R.A. (1984): The accuracy of fixation in lateral gaze and the problem of retinal slip. *Doc. Ophthalmol. 58*, 65–69.
Crone, R.A. (1988): A non-cyclopean diagram of binocular vision in strabismology. *Albrecht von Graefe's Arch. Klin. Exp. Ophthalmol. 226*, 113–116.
Crone, R.A. (1992): The history of stereoscopy. *Doc. Ophthalmol. 81*, 1–16.
Crone, R.A. (1992): *Licht–Kleur–Ruimte. De Leer van het Zien in Historisch Perspectief.* Bohn Stafleu Van Loghem, Houten/Zaventem.
Crone, R.A. (1999): *History of Color*. Kluwer Academic Publishers, Dordrecht, Boston, London.
Crone, R.A. (2000): Die Mondtäuschung und die scheinbare Grösse der Sonne. *Mitt. Julius-Hirschberg-Ges. Gesch. Augenheilk. 1*, 83–90.
Cronly-Dillon, R.G. (1991): The evolution of the eye. In: R.G. Cronly-Dillon (gen. ed.), *Vision and Visual Dysfunction*, Vol. 2. Macmillan Press, London.
Cyon, E. von (1901): Die physiologischen Grundlagen der Geometrie von Euklid. Eine Lösung des Raumproblems. *Pflügers Arch. Ges. Physiol., 85*, 576.
Dalen, J.T.W. van, van Rens, G.H. (1981): *The Brighter Side of Ophthalmology.* Holland Ophthalmic Publishing Center, Amersfoort.
Degenaar, M. (1996): *Molyneux's Problem: Three Centuries of Discussions on the Perception of Forms*. Kluwer Academic Publishers, Dordrecht.
Descartes, R. (1637): *Discours de la Méthode ... plus la Dioptrique, les Météores et la Géometrie*. Leiden.
Descartes, R. (1664): *Traité de l'Homme*. Paris.
De Valois, R.L., K.K. (1990): *Spatial Vision*. Oxford University Press, Oxford, New York.
Diderot, D. (1751): *Lettre sur les Aveugles, à l'Usage de ceux qui Voient*. Paris
Dieffenbach, J.F. (1839): Ueber das Schielen und die Heilung mittels Durchschneidung des inneren geraden Augenmuskels. *Med. Zeit. Verein. Heilk. Preussen 8*, 227–241.
Ditchburn, R.W. (1955): Eye movements in relation to retinal action. *Op. Acta 1*, 171–176.
Doesschate, G. ten (1930): Over den schijnbaren vorm van het hemelgewelf. *Nederl. Tijdschr. Geneesk. 74*, 748–754.
Donders, F.C. (1864): *On the Anomalies of Refraction and Accommodation of the Eye*. Repr. Erven F. Bohn, Haarlem.
Dowling, J.E. (1987): *The Retina*. Harvard University Press, Cambridge, Mass.

Dubois Reymond, E. (1872): Die Grenzen des Naturerkennens. In: Reden I. Berlin.

Duke-Elder, S. (1958–1976): *System of Ophthalmology. I. The Eye in Evolution* (1958). Henry Kimpton, London.

Edgerton Jr., S. (1975): *The Renaissance Rediscovery of Linear Perspective*. Icon Editions, Harper and Row, New York.

Einstein, A. (1917): *Ueber die spezielle und die allgemeine Relativitätstheorie gemeinverständlich.* Vieweg, Braunschweig.

Emmert, E. (1881): Grössenverhältnisse der Nachbilder. *Klin. Monatsbl. Augenheilk. 19*, 443–450.

Fischer, B., Boch, R. (1991): The Cerebral Cortex. In: R.G. Cronly-Dillon (gen. ed.), *Vision and Visual Dysfunction*, Vol. 8. Macmillan Press, London, pp. 227–296.

Frisby, J.P. (1979): *Seeing: Illusion, Brain and Mind*. University Press, Oxford.

Galileo (1623): *Il saggiatore*. Rome.

Gamov, G. (1940): Mr Tompkins in Wonderland. Repr. in: *Mr Tompkins in Paperback*. Press Syndicate of the University of Cambridge, Cambridge, U.S.A.

Gibson, J.J. (1950): *Perception of the Visual World*. Houghton Mifflin, Boston.

Grant, E. (1981): *Much Ado about Nothing. Theories of Space and Vacuum from the Middle Ages to the Scientific Revolution*. Cambridge University Press, Cambridge.

Greene, B. (1999): *The Elegant Universe: Superstrings, Hidden Dimensions, and the Quest for the Ultimate Theory.* Jonathan Cape, London.

Grüsser, O.-J., Landis, T. (1991): Visual agnosias and other disturbances of visual perception and cognition. In: R.G. Cronly-Dillon (gen. ed.), *Vision and Visual Dysfunction*, Vol. 12. Macmillan Press, London.

Guillemeau, J. (1585): *Traité des Maladies de l'Oeil, qui sont en Nombre de Cent Treize, ausquelles il est Sujet. Paris.*

Hammond, J.H. (1981): *The camera obscura, a cronicle*. Adam Hilger Ltd., Bristol.

Hartmann, N. (1947): *Neue Wege der Ontologie*. Repr. Wissenschaftliche Buchgesellschaft, Darmstadt, 1964.

Held, R. (1991): Development of binocular vision and stereopsis. In: R.G. Cronly-Dillon (gen. ed.), *Vision and Visual Dysfunction*, Vol. 9. Macmillan Press, London, pp. 170–180.

Helmholtz, H. von (1866): *Handbuch der physiologischen Optik*. Optik Voss, Heidelberg.

Hershenson, M. (1989): *The Moon Illusion*. Hillsdale, New York.

Hess, E. (1956): Plasticity in sensory-motor systems. *Sci. Amer. 195*, 84–94.

Holmes, G. (1918): Disturbances of vision by cerebral lesions. *Br. J. Ophthalmol. 2*, 353–384.

Hoorn, W. van (1972): *As Images Unwind. Ancient and Modern Theories of Visual Perception*. Amsterdam University Press, Amsterdam.

Hubel, D.H. (1988): *Eye, Brain and Vision*. Freeman & Co., New York.

Hubel, D.H., Wiesel, T. (1962): Receptive fields, binocular interaction and functional architecture in the cat's visual cortex. *J. Physiol.—London 165*, 106–154.

Jammer, M. (1954): *Concepts of Space. The History of Theories of Space in Physics*. Harvard University Press, Cambridge, Mass.

Jamnizer, W.W. (1568): *Perspectiva Corporum Regularium*. Vienna.

Jampel, R.S. (1959): Representation of the near response on the cerebral cortex of the macaque. *Amer. J. Ophthalmol. 48*, 573–581.

Javal, E. (1896): *Manuel du Strabisme*. Masson, Paris.

Julesz, B. (1964): Binocular depth perception without familiarity cues. *Science 145*, 356–362.

Julesz, B. (1971): *Principles of Cyclopean Perception*. University of Chicago Press, Chicago.

Kanizsa, G. (1955): Marzini quasi-percettivi in campi con stimulazione omogenea. *Rivist. Psycol. 49*, 7–30.

Kant, I. (1781): *Kritik der reinen Vernunft*. Riga.

Kaufman, L., Rock, I. (1962): The Moon Illusion. *Sci. Amer. 7*, 120–1130.
Kepler, J. (1604): *Ad Vitellionem Paralipomena, quibus Astronomiae pars Optica Traditur.* Frankfort.
Kepler, J. (1609): *Astronomia Nova.* Augsburg.
Klopp, H.W. (1951): Über Umgekehrt- und Verkehrtsehen. *Deuth. Z. Nervenheilk. 165*, 231–260.
Krol, J.D., van de Grind, W.A. (1980): The double-nail ilusion: Experiments on binocular vision with nails, needles, and pins. *Perception 9*, 651–669.
Kuffler, S.W. (1953): Neurons in the retina. *J. Neurophysiol. 16*, 37.
Lindberg, D.C. (1976): *Theories of Vision from Al-Kindi to Kepler.* University of Chicago Press, Chicago.
Lange, H. de (1952): Experiments on flicker and some calculations on an electrical analogue of the foveal system. *Physica, 18*, 935–950.
Locke, J. (1690): *An Essay Concerning Humane Understanding.* London.
Lotze, R.W. (1852): *Medizinische Psychlogie. Oder Physiologie der Seele.* Leipzig.
Mach, E. (1865). Ueber die Wirkung der räumlichen Vertheilung des Lichtreizes auf die Netzhaut. *Sitzb. Kaiserl. Akad. Wissensch., Math.-Naturwiss. Klasse, Wien, 52*, 303–322.
Marr, D. (1982): *Vision.* W.H. Freeman and Co., San Francisco.
Maxwell, J.C. (1873): *Treatise on Electricity and Magnetism.* Edinburgh.
Mesker, R.P. (1953): *De Optische Localisatie.* Swets en Zeitlinger, Amsterdam.
Mooney, A.J., Carey, P., Ryan, M., Bofin, P. (1965): Parasagittal parieto-occipital meningeoma. With visual hallucinations. *Amer. J. Ophthalmol., 13*, 238–246.
Motais, E. (1887): *Anatomie de l'Appareil Moteur de l'Oeil de l'Homme et des Vertébrés.* Delahaye et Lecrosnier, Paris.
Müller, J. (1826): *Zur vergleichenden Physiologie des Gesichtssinnes des Menschen und der Thiere.* Leipzig.
Nagel, T. (1974): What is it like to be a bat? *Phil. Rev. 83*, 435–451.
Newton, I. (1687): *Principia Mathematica Philosophiae Naturalis.* London.
Newton, I. (1704): *Opticks*, London. 4th corrected ed. 1730.
Østerberg, G. (1935): Topography of the layer of rods and cones in the human retina. *Acta Ophthalmol. Kbh. Suppl. 6.*
Pastore, N. (1971): *Selective History of Theories of Visual Perception.* Oxford University Press. New York, London.
Penfield, W.G., Rasmussen, T. (1952): *The Cerebral Cortex of Man.* Macmillan, New York.
Pettigrew, J.D. (1991): Evolution of Binocular Vision. In: R.G. Cronly-Dillon (gen. ed.), *Vision and Visual Dysfunction*, Vol. 2. Macmillan Press, London, pp. 271–283.
Poggio, G.F., Gonzalez, F., Krause, F. (1988): Stereoscopic mechanisms on monkey visual cortex: binocular correlation and disparity selectivity. *J. Neurosci. 8*, 4531.
Polyak, S. (1948): *The Retina.* The University of Chicago Press, Chicago.
Polyak, S. (1957): *The Vertebrate Visual System.* University of Chicago Press, Chicago.
Ratliff, F. (1965): *Mach Bands: Quantitative Studies on Neural Networks in the Retina.* Holden-Day, Inc., San Francisco, London, Amsterdam.
Reil, J.C. (1795): *Von der Lebenskraft.* Halle.
Rens, van (1981): *see* Dalen, van, van Rens (1981).
Roelofs, C.O. (1935): Die optische Lokalisation. *Arch. Augenheilk. 109*, 395.
Roelofs, C.O. (1960): Convergence and depth perception. *Acta Psychol. (Amst.) 17*, 193.
Rohault, J. (1672): *Traité de Physique.* Amsterdam.
Rose, A. (1973): *Vision: Human and Electronic.* Plenum Press, New York.
Sarnat, H.B., Netsky, M.G. (1974): *Evolution of the Nervous System.* Oxford University Press Inc., Oxford.

Schmidt, J.C., Gottlieb, M., Colemen, P., Smith, K.U. (1974): Reversal of retinal feedback of binocular eye movements in depth vision. *Amer. J. Optom. 51*, 382–399.
Schönbeck, G.L.J. (1998): *Sunbowl or Symbol: Models for the Interpretation of Heraclitus' Sun Notion.* Elixir Press, Amsterdam.
Smith, K.U. (1970): Inversion and delay of the retinal image: Feedback systems analysis of the classical problem of space perception. *Amer. J. Optom. and Arch. Amer. Acad. Optom, 47*, 175–204.
Snellen, H. (1862): *Letterproeven tot Bepaling der Gezigtsscherpte.* Utrecht.
Soemmering, S.T. (1786): *Ueber das Organ der Seele.* Göttingen.
Stenvers, H.W. (1945): *Contribution to the Diagnostics of Defects and Disorders of the Brain by Means of the Examination in the Fields of Vision and the Fields of Conjugate Movements to the Right and to the Left.* Noord-Hollandsche Uitgevers Maatschappij, Amsterdam.
Stone, L.S. (1947): Return of vision and functional polarization in the retinae of transplanted eyes. *Trans. Ophthalmol. Soc. UK 67*, 349–367.
Stratton, G.M. (1896): Some preliminary experiments in vision without inversion of the retinal image. *Psychol. Rev. 3*, 6611–6617.
Strong, D.S. (1979): *Leonardo and the Eye.* Garland Publishing, New York.
Trevarthen, C.B. (1968): Two mechanisms of vision in primates. *Psychol. Forsch. 31*, 299–337.
Trevarthen, C.B. (1970): Experimental evidence for a brain-stem contribution to visual perception in man. *Brain, Behav. Evol. 3*, 338–352.
Verheyen, F.J. (1961): A simple after-image method demonstrating the involuntary multidirectional eye movements during fixation. *Opt. Acta 8*, 309–311.
Vitello (1270): Optica (perspectiva). In: *Opticae Thesaurus Alhazeni Arabis Libri Septem . . . Item Vitellonis Thuringopoloni Libri* X. Risner, Basel, 1572. Reprint (1972) by Johnson Reprint Corporation, New York.
Voltaire, F.M. (1738): *Eléments de la Philosophie de Newton.* Amsterdam.
Wade, N.J. (1987): On the late invention of the stereoscope. *Perception 16*, 785–818.
Wade, N.J. (1998): *A Natural History of Vision.* M.I.T. Press, Cambridge, Mass.
Walls, G.L. (1942): *The Vertebrate Eye and its Adaptive Radiation.* Cranbrook Institute of Science, Bloomfield Hills, Mich.
Wertheim, Th. (1894): Über indirekte Sehschärfe. *Z. Psychol. Physiol. Sinnesorg. 7*, 172–183.
Westfall, R.S. (1980): *Never at Rest. A Biography of Isaac Newton.* Cambridge University Press, Cambridge.
Wheatstone, C. (1838): Contributions to the physiology of vision. *R. Soc. Philos. Trans. 128*, 371–394.
Witelo: see Vitello (1270).
Yarbus, A.L. (1967): *Eye Movements and Vision.* Plenum Press, New York.
Young, Th. (1802): On the theory of light and colours. *Phil. T. Roy. Soc. A*, 12–48.
Zeki, S. (1993): *A Vision of the Brain.* Blackwell Scientific Publications, Oxford.

INDEX